CW00410674

SEX

An Hachette UK Company
www.hachette.co.uk

First published in Great Britain in 2025
by Godsfield, an imprint of
Octopus Publishing Group Ltd
Carmelite House
50 Victoria Embankment
London EC4Y 0DZ
www.octopusbooks.co.uk

Copyright © Octopus Publishing Group
Ltd 2025

Distributed in the US by
Hachette Book Group
1290 Avenue of the Americas
4th and 5th Floors
New York, NY 10104

Distributed in Canada by
Canadian Manda Group
664 Annette St.
Toronto, Ontario, Canada M6S 2C8

ISBN 978-1-84181-605-0

A CIP catalogue record for this book is
available from the British Library.

Printed and bound in China

10 9 8 7 6 5 4 3 2 1

Publisher: Lucy Pessell
Designer: Isobel Platt
Editor: Feyi Oyesanya
Assistant Editor: Samina Rahman
Production Manager: Allison Gonsalves
Illustrations: Bárbara Malagoli

Ali Paul

SEX

**Everything everyone needs to
know about pleasure and play**

GODSFIELD

INTRODUCTION

8. WHAT IS SEX?

Pleasure, not positions • sex and safety • condoms • latex or polyurethane? • dental dams • how to love condoms • porn • keep it ethical • porn as inspo

17. BEFORE YOU BEGIN

Body positivity and body neutrality • sex positivity • how to build up to sex • talk • a word in your ear • tips for those in a relationship • lubrication • talking lube • types of lube • sex and drugs and alcohol • the power of touch • massage • handwork: gliding, kneading, deep pressure, percussion • pressure boost • the kidney meridian • more acupressure points for good sex • get fit for sex • your pelvic floor • PC exercises • sexercise

41. EXPLORE

Kissing • the body • the breasts and nipples • tit wanks or titty fucks • the vulva and vagina • exploring the vulva and vagina • watch • period play • acupressure points for period play • the penis and testicles • the P-spot • oral • if they have a clitoris • if they have a penis • deep-throat • power dynamics • anal play • rimming • penetration • anal positions • pegging • fisting • double penetration • deeper penetration • playing with the senses • sound • sight • lights on or off? • blindfolds • smell • taste • sex and food • food play

79. ORGASMS

Making it last • tantric bliss and edging • tantric tips for slowing down penetrative sex • if you have a penis • breathe • speeding up • coming together • tips for female orgasms • clitoral stimulation • squirting and female ejaculation • cervical orgasms • over and over • premature ejaculation • tips for delaying ejaculation • the squeeze technique for delaying ejaculation

97. VARIETY

Beyond the bedroom • water play • things to do in the shower • things to do in the bath • fast and furious • positions for fast sex • playtime • fun games to play • fantasy • role play • fantasies and relationships • toy box • good vibrations • toy hints and tips • kinks and fetishes • safe space • other ideas • edge-play and the dangers of extremes • bdsm • discipline, humiliation and degradation • submission and dominance • no pressure • bondage • before you tie up your partner • how to tie • pleasure and pain • impact play • adventurous vs power play • temperature play • breath play • safety • group sex • watching • events, clubs and parties • groups and relationships

INTRODUCTION

Are you ready to explore your sexuality, dissolve
all inhibitions and discover what feels right for
you and your partner?

Sometimes the furious pace of life, and inauthentic
and skewed representations of what sex is, and what
sexy is, make it difficult to remember that sex is all
about play.

Perhaps you take the anxieties and pressures of your
daily life, or negative thoughts about yourself to bed
with you? Maybe you've never felt able to discover –
let alone communicate to a partner about – what turns
you on? Are you in a long-term relationship and don't
want the magic to fade? If your sex life has got stuck
in a rut, you'll find plenty of ideas for spicing things up
and lots of ways of rediscovering your own sensuality
and sense of fun – and that of the person, or people,
you are with.

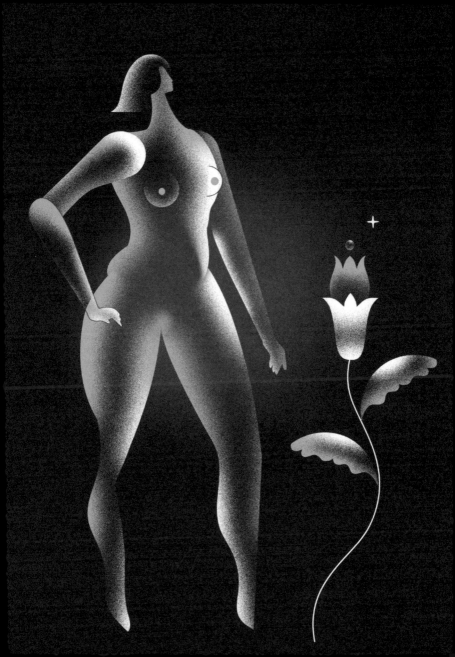

WHAT IS SEX?

Foreplay was conventionally thought of as being whatever form of arousal came before penetrative sex – and specifically, one penis–one vagina penetration. Kissing, licking, fingering...anything that was the preamble to 'the big act', or the no-frills fast track to orgasm. But that puts penetrative sex on a pedestal it often isn't – and doesn't always deserve to be – on.

First, sex doesn't have to be penetrative at all. 'Outercourse' is a very real thing for a lot of people and they receive as much pleasure from it as others do from intercourse. Second, penetrative sex isn't the surest way to the most intense orgasms – ask anyone who's had a clitoral or nipple orgasm. And third, you don't need one person with a penis and one person with a vagina in order to have sex – penetrative or otherwise.

It's helpful to think of what convention calls 'foreplay' as something that brings both body and mind to an enhanced state of arousal. And something that doesn't have to come before anything else. It's just play.

Masturbation, foreplay, outercourse and penetrative sex are all forms of sex and sex is play. It's the delicious exploration of bodies – entire bodies, not just the genitals – and opens the door to total body sensation and arousal.

This book is aimed at everyone regardless of gender, sexuality or how you identify yourself. We refer to 'your partner' frequently but that could well be two people, not a singular partner. We simply use 'your partner' to avoid multiple(s) throughout the book. And if you're playing solo, this book is for you too. Sex doesn't have to involve anyone other than you. Too often we dismiss solo masturbation as 'getting ourselves off', or diminish it as a quick 'wank' or 'jerk off' when we could be taking our masturbation slowly and our pleasure to new levels.

PLEASURE, NOT POSITIONS

This book is all about pleasure and how to get the most out of sex. We sometimes suggest what might be good positions if you want to try something for the first time but we're not going to give you our top 10 of the best positions ever because everybody – literally 'every body', is different.

Don't stress about forcing yourself into a pose that's going to be so uncomfortable to hold that you can't feel any pleasure. Cramp just isn't sexy. Why worry about being too heavy to straddle a lighter partner when you could just bend over? Don't go for deep penetration if it's going to cause you pain or discomfort. If you're squeezed into a toilet cubicle, it's probably not the time to attempt the Piledriver...you get the gist.

If you want to expand your repertoire, there's a wealth of information out there but always think first about your and your partner's bodies and their limits – pleasure comes first.

SEX AND SAFETY

This book is intended to offer tips, advice and techniques to people who are safe and secure no matter what sort of relationship they are in – be they committed and loving, spontaneous and anonymous, adventurous and one-off, or anything in between. Whatever the nature of the encounter, the consent and emotional and physical wellbeing of all parties is a non-negotiable.

The tips and ideas offered are for inspiration only and should not be interpreted as 'normal', necessary nor anticipated in any form of relationship. Positive, healthy and rewarding sex requires mutual trust, respect and appreciation of each other's feelings, bodies and boundaries.

If you feel anxious or vulnerable during sex, stop. You should never feel pressured to try anything that you are not comfortable with or let an individual or group persuade you that you should.

'Safe words' often come up in chat about kinky or power play but they're there for everyone, all of the time. Establishing safe words when engaging in sex with another person or people allows you to establish clear boundaries and communicate when you want to stop. If you are engaging in kink play, do not choose words such as 'stop' or 'no' as kink often involves consent to the fantasy of non-consent and you may not be understood.

! However, in all other circumstances, 'no' and 'stop' mean 'no' and 'stop'.

! Never pressure another person to engage in any activity that makes them physically or emotionally uncomfortable. If you are considering engaging in or consenting to something that you are unsure of, always seek advice or further information from a range of trusted resources that consider and champion safety, diversity and inclusion. And then take time to consider that advice and information and what it might mean to you.

! If you or anyone you know is in a situation where they feel unsafe, unsupported or at risk of harm seek immediate help.

CONDOMS

SAFE AND SEXY

If you're uncommitted, restless and sexually adventurous or just starting a new relationship, we share a few tips about how to make using a condom both fun and sexy.

Condoms are about 98 per cent effective in protecting against unwanted pregnancy and 85 per cent effective in protecting against sexually transmitted infections but not everyone loves them. Among the most common complaints are that they're uncomfortable, they reduce sensation or it's just plain awkward to take a break from play to put one on.

Latex or polyurethane?

Latex condoms need to be used with water-based lubricants such as KY jelly, as oil can damage the latex. If you're allergic to latex, or it causes a burning sensation, try condoms made of polyurethane. These tend to be stronger and are safe to use with most lubricants, including oils.

DENTAL DAMS

Dental Dams are a type of protection specifically designed for oral sex. They're usually made of latex and despite being called 'dental dams' they're not worn in the mouth but instead cover the vulva, vagina or anus to form a barrier between the area and the mouth. They are intended to protect against STIs but are only effective if used properly so always read the instructions.

HOW TO LOVE CONDOMS

- Experiment with different brands and use plenty of the appropriate lube.
- Go shopping for special condoms. Browse in sex shops or specialist online outlets for something different. Try coloured or flavoured ones (although avoid these if you're prone to yeast infections).
- Condoms with ribs, tendrils or bobbles on them are designed to stimulate the vaginal and anal walls and may stimulate the G-spots.
- Accept that although the sensation of sex with a condom might feel different, you can find other ways to stimulate you and your partner during sex.
- Don't let breaking off from play to put on a condom spoil the mood – make it a part of it. Watch your partner put one on, or put it on for them. Try massaging a drop of lube onto the tip of the penis or toy with a finger first. Make rolling it down the shaft part of the masturbation – use your lips as well as your fingers to smooth it down. Try to put one on using your mouth alone – no teeth!

! If you're taking a toy or penis from the anus to the vagina, remove the condom and put on a new one.

PORN

Porn is a tricky subject as it's fraught with issues such as the health and wellbeing of its subjects, whether it has an overwhelmingly negative impact on emotional development and relationships, whether it damages our self-esteem and whether it normalizes degradation or objectification.

There is no right answer and if you are unsure about watching porn then research different points of view thoroughly and spend time assessing whether it might be right for you. While it is common that people watch porn, that is not the same as saying it is 'normal' to watch porn so whether you do or don't, you're normal and should not be made to feel otherwise.

KEEP IT ETHICAL

Until relatively recently, most porn was made by heterosexual men for heterosexual men – it used to be assumed that women weren't turned on by sex on film, and homosexual, transexual or any form of queer porn was very much an underground subsect. Now, mainstream porn sites host a growing amount and variety of content that more accurately reflects society and sex and body positivity.

'Ethical porn' refers to porn made fairly (everyone receives a share of the money), with the full consent of all parties (the actors but also everyone on set), with everyone's safety ensured, and with real world sex and real world bodies included.

OK, so this is a bit of a generalization, but trad porn since the 90s has usually featured a slim woman with perky tits and no pubic hair having a fake orgasm as she's being drilled, nailed or stretched by one or several massive cocks. Ethical porn is more likely to feature diverse body types, people of any gender and real pleasure. There may or may not be pubic hair and body hair. Tits, vulvas, penises and anuses will come in a variety of colours, sizes and shapes, and they'll squelch, squirt and smear all the right fluids.

Things are changing fast but if you're unsure where to start, it's best to make a specific search for 'ethical porn'.

PORN AS INSPO

A lot of mainstream porn still leads with the degradation or dehumanizing of (usually) women, and until more recently, it was impossible to tell whether it involved consent, or was coercive and abusive. Increasingly, even mainstream pornsites are hosting content that features degrading or abusive acts that begin and end with interviews with the (usually) women featured in which they clearly state their consent, and describe their pleasure afterwards.

Keep in mind that a lot of the more degrading or extreme acts such as submission, gang bangs and fisting have hit the mainstream via porn and while they're undeniably enjoyable for some, they're still carrying a lot of misogynistic baggage. ALL play must always be for the pleasure and gratification of ALL parties.

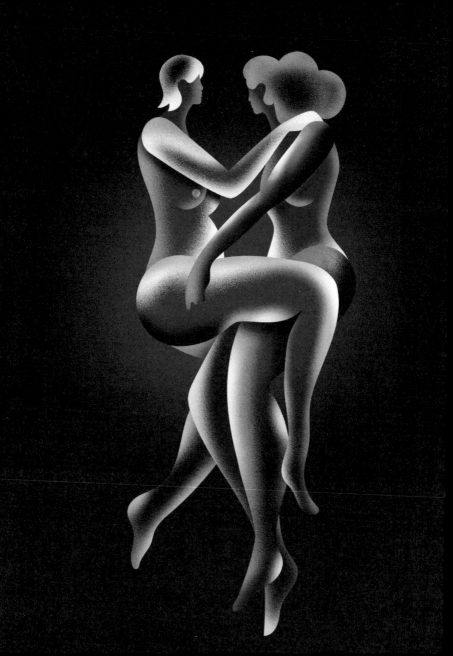

BEFORE
YOU BEGIN

BODY POSITIVITY AND BODY NEUTRALITY

Body positivity is about loving and celebrating your body, or parts of your body, unconditionally and regardless of its shape, size, colour or myriad of attributes.

Body neutrality is less about loving your body and more about accepting and appreciating it for its function, not form. So rather than saying 'I love my beautiful legs' you'd be more likely to say 'my legs are strong and support me as I run'.

People in both camps are still prone to insecurities, hang-ups and negativity about parts of their bodies but generally, their positivity or neutrality outweighs that. Anxiety about our bodies can wreak havoc with our mood, focus and senses and make us far less likely to free ourselves of inhibitions during sex.

If you hate that roll of belly fat and are only thinking about trying to hide it, you're going to be limiting yourself to 'flattering' positions rather than those that will open your eyes and G-, C-, P- and A-spots to new pleasures, you'll be tightening your muscles and tensing your body in ways that inhibit sensations in others, and your mind will be focused on that negative thought and not on your pleasure or your partner's.

Accepting or loving your own body will give you the confidence – emotional and physical – to let go, enjoy sex and experience pleasure in all-new ways. If you're concerned about not conforming to a beauty ideal, take some time to explore the thinking behind body positivity and neutrality. Stop scrolling through social media accounts that only support a single-gaze view of bodies and proactively seek out different voices and representations. Do literally anything other than hate your body.

If you've had sex with two people, it's unlikely that both of them would have had exactly the same body type, the same shape of penis or the same labial folds, the same scent, the same colour anus, the same type of body hair in exactly the same place. But chances are, you found them attractive, right? Well chances are, it's a case of right back atcha.

SEX POSITIVITY

Sex positivity is, broadly, anything that promotes the
enjoyment of sex regardless of gender, sex, sexuality,
medicine or repressive cultural norms.

Sex positivity was initially championed by the feminist
movements of the 1960s-80s but has become a movement
that encompasses all sexes, genders and identities.

Sex positivity is all about exploring sex, sexuality and gender
and whatever turns you on – to hell with old-fashioned and
heteronormative, toxic taboos. It's about breaking down often
misogynistic, patriarchal or oppressive views and allowing
people to explore their bodies and others' bodies without shame.

Own a vagina but want to know how it feels to thrust a
'penis' into your male partner? Do it. Own a penis that has
only ever entered vaginas but want to know how it feels to be
penetrated? Do it. Own a clitoris but want to flick a clitoris
with your tongue? Do it. Want to watch while other people
lick and suck and penetrate others? Do it.

And enjoy it all. That's sex positivity.

HOW TO
BUILD UP TO SEX

For some people, having sex or making love is easy. For others,
it's difficult to give all of themselves sexually if they don't feel
totally secure.

Someone who wants to give their partner an emotionally safe place
in which to let go and express their sexuality without inhibitions will
understand that sex begins way before you get to the bedroom. It
lies in the way you speak to each other, look at each other and touch
each other. That doesn't necessarily mean that your manner should
be sexually loaded, but it should express affection, appreciation and
(if you're in a committed relationship) your love.

TALK

Communication is the single most important key to great sex.
Whether it's to find out what your partner likes, how to turn
each other on, set boundaries and limits, or express and allay
fears or anxieties, being able to talk about sex is crucial.

Author Isabel Allende wrote: 'For women, the best aphrodisiacs
are words. The G-spot is in the ears. He who looks for it below
there is wasting his time.' Although Allende referred to 'women',
the same is true for many people regardless of how they identify.

A WORD IN YOUR EAR

- **Make eye contact** and **compliment** your partner. Get specific – perhaps it's a particular freckle, the glint in their eye, the way they part their lips.
- **Whisper into their ears** – the ears are an erogenous zone that can be stimulated by sound and breath. Lick their earlobes as you whisper.
- **Ask questions** – what do they like? What do they want? What do they want you to do?
- **Talk dirty** – whether in person or sexting, build anticipation. Tell them what you want them to do to you, tell them what you want to do to them. If you've already had sex with them, tell them what you loved about last time, then describe what's going to happen next time.
- During sex, **keep talking**. Tell your partner how good what they're doing feels and tell them how good they look. Tell them how hard or wet you are, or how close to orgasm you are.
- In the English language, it's common to use sex words to express anger and as insults. In other (arguably less-repressed) cultures, sex words are used only for sex. To some of us, it feels wrong to use what are often thought of as obscenities to express pleasure. **Try using words as they were originally intended** and feel their erotic power – call fucking 'fucking', the penis 'dick' or 'cock', your vagina your 'pussy' and yes, we're going there – your 'cunt'.

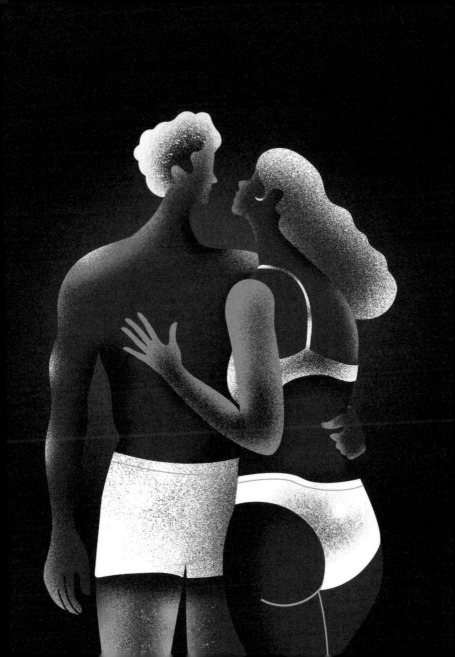

TIPS FOR THOSE IN A RELATIONSHIP
WHERE THE MAGIC HAS FADED

Feeling loved is one of the best aphrodisiacs
available to us.

- Ask your partner about themself and don't forget to listen while they tell you.
- **Touch them a lot** – hug them, stroke their back, kiss the top of their head.
- **Pay them small attentions** to show that you think of them when you aren't together – phone to ask how they are or give them bizarre little presents that will touch their heart.
- **Tell your partner you love them** and care about them deeply. There's nothing more intoxicating than hearing this. If your partner asks for reassurance, avoid sarcasm: 'Well, I wouldn't still be with you if I didn't, would I?' only ever sounds like a put-down, and if they're feeling insecure it will make them more anxious still.
- **Talk about your commitment** and make plans together. To affirm that your relationship has a positive future is a real morale booster.
- Often, as we settle into committed relationships, cute – or even knowingly goofy – names and nicknames creep into our vocabulary. Consider dropping words such as 'willy' or 'boobs' for **something filthier** such as 'cock', 'dick' or 'pussy' before and during sex.
- Offer to give them a **massage** – relaxing or erotic.

LUBRICATION

Sex is all about movement – rubbing, sliding, slipping, pushing, licking, stroking – and none of these can happen without lubrication. It's time to dispel the myth that dryness = you don't want sex. Some vaginas and rectums are awash with secretions, while others are more dry – there's no 'normal' here.

- Vaginal dryness is often a natural accompaniment to menopause or breastfeeding but it can also be caused by contraceptive pills, antidepressants and a host of other things.
- Although the anus does have lubrication glands, anal sex often requires plenty of lubrication to avoid friction, fissures and tears.
- Dryness is completely normal but it can make sex less comfortable so never, ever feel embarrassed or ashamed to reach for the lube.

TALKING LUBE

Be confident! Remember that sex is all about pleasure. If you're still worried and are beginning a relationship with a new partner, discuss the joys of lube before you get down to business. Talk about it on an occasion when you feel close but are not yet ready to embark on the sexual side of your relationship.

TYPES OF LUBE

It's important to be able to talk about lube to establish what will be safe for you and your partner – some people are allergic to key ingredients in both natural and synthetic lubes. Broadly speaking, lube breaks down into 3 types: water-based, silicone-based and all-natural oils.

- **Silicone-based lube** is great for a velvety smooth glide and is longer-lasting than water-based alternatives. Silicone-based lubes tend to be pH-neutral and are unlikely to interfere with the vagina's pH levels. Most silicone lubes are safe to use with condoms but don't use them with silicone toys as it can damage them.
- **Water-based lube** gives a light and natural sensation that's easy to wash off – but conversely that means they aren't suitable for water play. Most are safe to use with all types of condoms and toys but many contain ingredients such as glycerine which may irritate skin and can trigger yeast infections.
- **Oil-based lubes** are long-lasting and can be a great natural alternative to consider but they are not compatible with latex condoms. Be aware that they are associated with yeast infections and can stain fabrics. Coconut oil, and sweet almond oil are both excellent lubricants and a natural alternative to proprietary brands. The advantage of sweet almond oil is that it has only a faintly sweet and nutty taste, which does not spoil the flavour of human skin or juices. It is colourless and non-sticky, but in addition to the previous precautions, do be careful to check that your partner doesn't have a nut allergy!

SEX AND DRUGS AND ALCOHOL

- Everyone knows that alcohol loosens the tongue and the inhibitions – but though it enlivens at first, it's technically still a depressant. A little too much and you'll be drowsy – more than that and the urge and ability to have sex might leave altogether.
- Recreational drugs, like alcohol, induce a chemical high followed by an emotional low, while dreamy cannabis encourages sleep, rather than great sex. Ask yourselves whether it's sex you want, or each other. It can be a lonely and alienating experience if you get the feeling your partner's deriving their pleasure from taking a drug instead of just from being with you.
- Both drugs and alcohol can reduce our inhibitions too far and leave us vulnerable.
- If you smoke, you should be aware that nicotine reduces the production of nitric oxide, which is the body's main chemical messenger that triggers the pumping of blood to the penis.

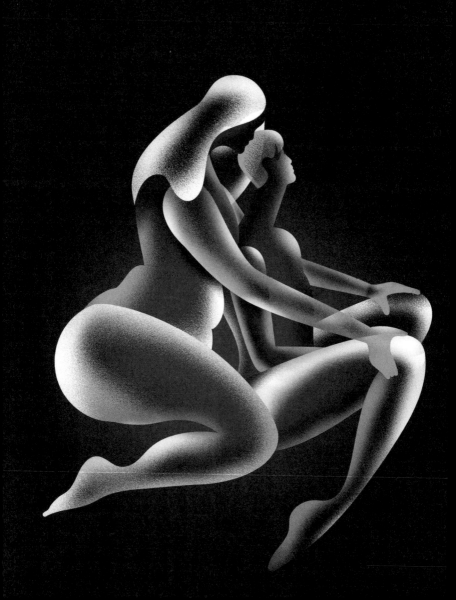

THE POWER
OF TOUCH

For some people, sex itself triggers stress for a whole host of reasons including body image and performance anxiety. If that's the case for you, it's worth exploring those feelings and finding ways to improve your relationship with sex but you might find that relieving stress in your body alleviates some of what's going on in your head.

Stress and anxiety are enemies of sex and even when we think our mind is clear, our bodies are often holding on to our angst and tension. The more problems or pressure in our lives, the greater the tension that accumulates in all of the parts of our bodies that could be priming us for pleasure.

If you're carrying stress in your body, you'll likely have muscle knots or will be tensing your neck, back or limbs to protect them. Relaxing your body is a great way to prepare you for the physical and emotional experience of sex.

MASSAGE

Touch is one of the most intimate modes of communication, and massage is one of the oldest forms of healing and relaxation. A massage signifies total acceptance of the body, transmits affirmation and boosts self-esteem – it can touch the emotions as well as the body and will help to alleviate both mental and physical stress.

Massage is also a great way to observe your partner's body and to tune in to each other physically and emotionally before there is any pressure to perform.

Relaxation and sex go hand in hand and massage offers many opportunities to discover erogenous zones you never knew you had – even the most innocuous foot or hand massage can quickly turn erotic.

MASSAGE TIPS

- Remove jewellery and keep nails short and smooth.
- Make sure your partner is warm enough. Cover the part of the body you are not working on.
- Use massage oil to lubricate their skin.
- Warm the oil in your hands first – don't pour it directly on to the skin.
- Be gentle and try to keep at least one hand on the body at all times.
- Minimize conversation so that you are communicating through touch.

HANDWORK

The laying on of hands is comforting, reassuring, calming and healing. There are four basic massage strokes: gliding, kneading, deep pressure and percussion.

Technique 1: Gliding

- **Glide your hands smoothly and rhythmically** over your partner's skin. This soothing stroke is ideal to use at the beginning and end of a session: the broad strokes 'join up' the body after you have worked on specific areas.
- **Vary the firmness** and speed of your strokes, and experiment with applying most pressure from the heels or palms of your hands.
- **Draw wavy lines** on your partner's skin, opening out and closing your fingers.
- **Try a light pressure** with the fingertips. This is quite difficult to do without tickling, so wait until your partner is fully relaxed.
- **Use alternate strokes** – let one hand follow the other, skimming across the skin as if you were brushing crumbs towards yourself.
- **Make big circles** with your hands, letting one hand follow the other. This is a very good stroke for centring the body and banishing mental stress.
- Kneeling at your partner's head, glide both your hands down the back together, pushing quite firmly, then draw them up again.

Technique 2: Kneading

This is a vigorous stroke and one that gives instant relief, transforming the body under your hands from sluggish and fatigued to light and energetic. The key lies in rhythmic repetition, which builds up a momentum that is almost hypnotic.

> Choose a fleshy area on which to practise, such as the buttocks. Put your palms flat on your partner's body with fingers together and your hands pointing at 45° degrees towards each other.

> **Make small circles** with your hands, moving them up and outwards in turn, following each other.

> Now add the **thumb movement** – every time your hand moves up and out, your thumb moves separately behind it, grasping the flesh and pushing it firmly along, as if you were kneading bread. You can feel the tensed muscles softening under your hands as you work.

> There are a few variations on this stroke. **Wringing** is where the hands work simultaneously in opposite directions. For **pulling**, sit on one side of your partner, reach across to the other side of the back and pull the flesh firmly towards you with alternate hands. A third variation is to **nip** the flesh between fingers and thumb, tugging and then releasing. Use alternate hands.

Technique 3: Deep pressure

> Apply **deep pressure** with your thumbs, but wait until your partner is fully relaxed, or it might hurt.

> **Press firmly** into the flesh with the balls of your thumbs, making little circles and pushing the skin away from you. Put your weight behind the movement.

> Move across areas of particular tension, working with both thumbs together or using them alternately.

Technique 4: Percussion

Invigorating rather than sensual, this is a stroke to use on fleshy parts of the body to get your partner relaxed. In percussion, always allow the hand to relax at the wrist before contact so that you are using just the weight of your hand rather than the force of your whole arm. Keep up a strong hypnotic rhythm – think of the steady drumming of heavy rain.

- **One-handed percussion**: as your left hand glides over your partner's skin, pound it repeatedly with the weight of your right fist (or the other way round).
- **Two-handed percussion**: keep up a loose drumming rhythm, working with alternate fists. Work lightly on sensitive areas, trying percussion with the tips of your index fingers.
- **Hacking**: work with palms facing each other, hands flat, fingers together. This technique is good for use on the buttocks, thighs and calves, but it could be painful elsewhere.

PRESSURE BOOST

Try a regular massage of specific pressure points to boost your sexual energy. The Japanese therapy of shiatsu is based on the philosophy and medical theory of acupuncture.

Shiatsu works with the flow of energy called *ki* that runs through the body in channels known as meridians. By working pressure points along these meridians, blockages can be dissolved and the flow of energy released.

THE KIDNEY MERIDIAN

Working some of the body's pressure points can increase and strengthen the flow of their sexual energy.

Sexuality is governed, for the most part, by the kidney meridian. The kidney pressure points, or *tsubos*, are found about one thumb's width, or *cun*, on either side of the spine, level with the space between the second and third lumbar vertebrae. Work both left and right *tsubos* at once.

You know when you have found the *tsubo* when your thumb nestles into a small hollow. If it feels full of energy, with strong muscle tone or a sharp tender feeling, keep your thumb on the spot, or make small circling or pumping motions until you feel the energy relax. If energy is lacking and the *tsubo* feels empty and needy, hold your thumb in the spot until you feel the energy return.

MORE ACUPRESSURE POINTS
FOR GOOD SEX

- **Kidney Back Transporting Point:** 1.5 *cun* to the sides of the spine, level with the space between the second and third lumbar vertebrae. Excellent for lack of sexual desire in either sex.
- **Greater Stream:** right between the ankle bone and the Achilles tendon. Treats lack of vitality and sexual energy.
- **Gate of Life:** between the second and third lumbar vertebrae. Boosts vitality and libido.
- **Gate to Original Ki:** 3 *cun* below the navel – good for fatigue and boosting libido.

GET FIT FOR SEX

This isn't about *looking* fit – no 'beach body ready'
chat here, thanks – this is about *getting* fit.

Sex is often touted as the best exercise ever, and exercise and
fitness make for better sex. Keeping in good shape means
you have more energy, alertness, flexibility and stamina.
This in turn builds confidence, body neutrality, and a better
relationship between body and mind.

Science suggests we should do at least 30 minutes of exercise
per day or vigorous aerobic exercises one hour every other
day. In one study, 50-year-old male office workers with
erection problems did this for nine months – by which time
they were having sex 30 per cent more often than they had
been when they started. A control group walked for one hour
every other day – with no recorded benefits to their sex lives.

YOUR PELVIC FLOOR

If regular exercise isn't your thing and you do nothing
else, keep the pelvic floor strong.

The pelvic floor is a network of muscles that support the organs of
the pelvis – the bladder, genitals and anus. You can feel where it is
by contracting the muscles at the front that would stop a flow of
urine, and those at the back that would stop a bowel movement.

Toning these very same muscles – the pubococcygeus, or PC for
short – is a sure way to improve sex and can increase the intensity
of the female orgasm. Far less research has been conducted into
the advantages of PC exercises for males with penises but they are
believed to have a positive effect on sexual function, premature
ejaculation and stress incontinence.

- In all genders, age can affect the tautness and elasticity of
  the PC but there are other factors too, including bladder
  and bowel issues.
- In females, the muscles of the pelvic floor are often
  seriously weakened by childbirth, particularly if labour
  has been long and difficult. The result is that the vagina
  loses some of its snug and responsive elasticity and
  may feel slack during sex. Exercising these muscles
  regularly helps keep them toned, which in turn improves
  their elasticity.
- In males, the PC can be weakened by prostate issues and
  can cause erectile dysfunction.

PC EXERCISES

Keep your PC muscles supple with Kegel exercises (so called after their inventor). The advantage with these exercises is that you can do them anywhere, at any time, without anyone knowing – in the bath, in the office, on the bus...

> Keep the rest of your body relaxed and breathe slowly and steadily as you perform the exercise.

> Repeatedly contract the PC muscles as strongly as you can for 5 seconds, then slowly relax them. When you find this easy, work up to contracting the muscles for 10 seconds.

> Unless you have recently given birth, you should aim to perform 150 contractions a day.

> Vary the exercise: start with the front, bladder connected muscles, then move on to the back, anus-connected muscles. Or alternate between the two.

- Weighted Kegel balls (or Ben Wa balls) can be inserted into the vagina and left in place for 2-3 hours at a time.
- ! Never insert Kegel balls designed for the vagina into the anus – use plugs and balls designed for anal insertion.
- After childbirth, exercising twice a day for 20 minutes can help the muscles recover and prevent further weakening.
- Males can develop a stronger and more sensitive erection by 'waving the wand'. Sit on the edge of the bed. Locate the muscles that move your penis up and down and from side to side, and flex them for about 10 minutes every day.
- Flex your muscles during penetrative sex.

SEXERCISE

Exercise raises the blood levels of hormones involved in the chemistry of arousal – it makes you want sex more urgently, more often. So why not exercise together?

WORK OUT THEN MAKE OUT

- If you have an exercise bench, use it for robust sexercises in which you thrust against one another. Your partner lies on their back and pushes by holding on to support bars, while you stand between their legs.
- Go running together, pacing yourselves well against each other, then take a hot shower together afterwards, and enjoy endorphin-fuelled and invigorated sex.
- Dancing is an amazing form of energetic, fluid and inherently sexy exercise. Combine it with performing a striptease, or just undress each other to music. Try carrying positions for having sex to music.

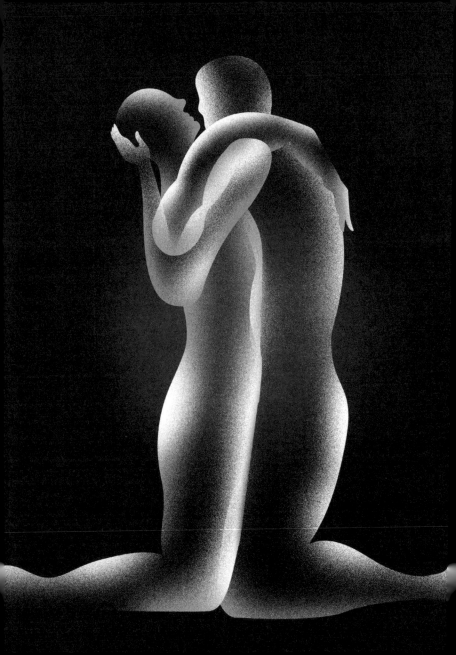

EXPLORE

To get the most fun out of sex you need to explore both your own and your partner's erotic responses. Everyone has their own special erogenous zones and preferred rituals and positions. Tantalizing and accommodating these parts of you are vital to great sex, but don't forget that you can add interest, spice and variety through experimentation.

Erogenous zones are those parts of our bodies that produce sexual pleasure when stimulated. No body is the same and many of us don't know how many we have because they're yet to be explored. That's why play – solo or otherwise – is so important.

Giving parts of your partner's body your full attention, or receiving their attention to parts of yours is a powerful turn-on.

- **Study the sensitivity of the erogenous zones** in minute detail to familiarize yourself with their unique desires and needs. You might discover that the heat of their breath on the back of your knee, or the flick of a tongue along your inner arm drives you wild. You might be the first person to have slid a knuckle along your partner's perineum or grazed the inside of their wrist with your lips.
- **Experiment with different types of friction** with your tongue, fingers and genitals to discover the best way to arouse them. Then investigate ways of varying stimulation so that you can pace arousal. Control of timing is the secret of long-lasting, satisfying play.

KISSING

Don't roll your eyes and flip through the book to find 'G-spot'. Kissing is one of the greatest turn-ons but one many people rush in order to get to the sexy bits. The thing is, kissing stimulates the sexy bits.

- **Be imaginative** with your lips and tongue. Use their mobility and suppleness to communicate your feelings.
- **Pay attention** to the corners of your partner's mouth with your tongue, probing gently inside the mouth to echo the feeling of a penis or toy penetrating a vagina or anus.
- Try gently **sucking** on your partner's tongue or lower lip.
- Who takes the lead? Try leading yourself or tune into your partner's kiss. Or play passive and allow yourself to be kissed – this can feel particularly good for someone who usually plays more dominant.
- Have your partner open their mouth and bare the tongue, then lick across it with generous broad strokes from corner to corner – an especially arousing kiss.
- **Stimulate** the nerves that run along the thinnest part of the upper lip by grazing your tongue across them.
- What to do with your hands? Cradle your partner's face, support their neck, stroke their hair. Some people are driven wild by a finger gently inserted into their mouth along with a tongue.

THE BODY

For the most intense, languorous sex play, the breasts and genitals should be the rapturous end of a long journey across and around the body.

Skimming unexpectedly over the usual erogenous zones builds erotic anticipation, passing intense feeling on to the next part, and turning your whole body into a finely tuned pleasure zone.

- **The Hair** The scalp is full of nerve endings and stimulating them sends tingles down your spine. Apply gentle pressure to the scalp with your fingers before gently pulling them through the hair. Some people like to have their hair tugged or pulled during play.
- **The Ear** Some people love having their earlobes nibbled and sucked. Some love to have their ears licked, with the tongue slowly swirling round the contours of the ear flap and flicking down inside.
- **The Knee** The knees are erotically sensitive but an often neglected part of the body. Graze the back of the knee with your lips or run your fingernails across it.
- **The Navel** Lick with the flat of your tongue in broad strokes, sweeping in a clockwise direction around the navel and circling inwards. Then hold your partner's buttocks with one hand, pressing the heel of the hand very firmly into the perineum and pulling upwards, and dance the tip of your tongue all around and over the belly button, exploring every tiny crevice. Hit the right nerve here and you'll send a tingling sensation streaking right down to the genitals.

- **The Buttocks** There's lots of scope on this fleshy part for vigorous activity, such as kneading, playful smacks, sucking and nibbling – but don't neglect the sensitivity of the skin. Stroke the buttocks ever so lightly with your palm and fingertips, trailing your hand in lazy circles around their curves.
- **The feet** can be really ticklish so start with a slow and deliberate massage.

> Hold one foot in both hands and work with your thumbs, feeling around all the bones on the top of the feet, from the base of the toes up towards the ankle. You should be applying firm pressure and avoiding tickly, feathery motions.

> Hold the foot up, support it under the calf or ankle and press deeply on the sole with your thumb or the heel of the other hand, working round the contours of the foot. Lower the foot and work on the toes. Work on each toe, moving with small twiddlings of finger and thumb that feel all the tiny bones from the base to the tip. Then pull off at the tip, as if you were pulling off socks with toes in them.

> Try sucking your partner's toes one by one.

> Experiment with using the your partner's big toe to penetrate you – some people find this very erotic. Short nails and smooth skin, please. It adds a new dimension to games of footsie under the table.

THE BREASTS AND NIPPLES

Observe your partner's breasts during sex. Each person reacts differently, but many develop a flush that spreads from above the waist right across their chest. The areola – the dark disc around the nipple – may swell or get darker. Both male and female nipples can be extremely sensitive and yes, nipplegasms are a real thing for some people.

- The upper breast is generally more sensitive than the lower breast.
- **Cup and lift** the breasts in both hands, massaging underneath them with a gentle circular motion.
- Work in **tantalizing swirls** with your tongue around the nipple, focusing on the areola and the sensitive skin in the upper third of the breast.
- Try **gentle kneading** and experimental nibbling.
- In many people, the nipples become erect when they're aroused. If the nipple isn't erect, run the flat of your tongue across it in slow, broad strokes.
- **Squeeze**, **gently twist** or **massage** the nipples with your fingers.
- **Swirl your tongue** around the areola and then quickly poke the nipple with the tip of your tongue.
- For some people, the nipples are so sensitive that it's possible to experience a 'nipplegasm'.

TIT WANKS OR TITTY FUCKS

The breasts can be used to masturbate the penis by squeezing it between them. It's a form of non-penetrative play (technically known as mammary intercourse) that's pleasurable for the giver and the receiver. While the receiver thrusts between the breasts, the giver can stimulate their nipples.

- Use plenty of lube to increase the stimulation.
- Straddling gives the receiver control: the giver lies on their back with the receiver either straddling their chest, or straddling their head facing their toes (this presents an opportunity for rimming).
- For the giver to be in control, the receiver sits on the edge of the bed with the giver kneeling between their legs.
- People with smaller breasts may find this kind of play a little more difficult and may need to use their mouth or hands at intervals but it's still an incredible turn-on to have your assets centre stage.

! Menstruation and breastfeeding can make breasts and nipples tender. Lightly stroke swollen breasts on the less sensitive underside.

! If your partner has had a breast implant, sensitivity won't be impaired, but take care in moving the breasts. Avoid vigorous handling and use feathery caresses with fingers or tongue.

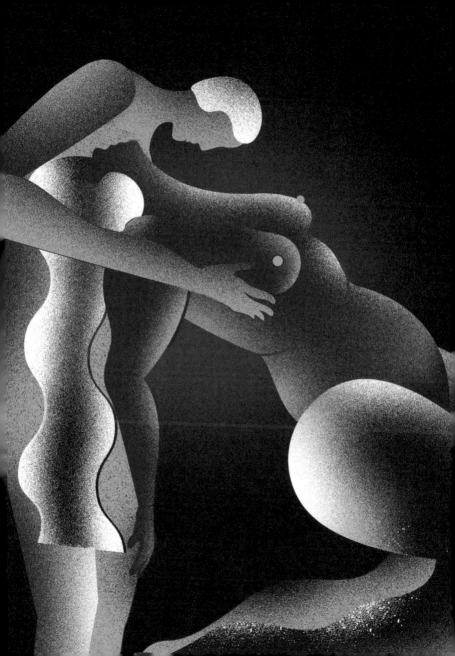

THE VULVA AND VAGINA

THE VULVA

The vulva is the name for the external parts of the female genitalia including the clitoris, the labia and the vaginal opening. The vagina is the internal passage.

Although the clitoris is usually the most sensitive part of the vulva, it's often best left until last.

EXPLORING THE VULVA AND VAGINA

> Explore your partner's vulva and vagina as if you have never seen or felt one before.

> Begin by gently stroking the flats of your palms across their pubic bone and upper thighs. Gently part their legs and put their feet on your shoulders.

> Stroke the whole area, just very lightly, then press your open lips to the skin of the upper thigh and breathe warm air on to it, circling the vulva and eventually homing in on it. Don't use your tongue.

> Your partner should now be feeling warm, relaxed and very responsive. Part the labia and very gently explore the shape of the vulva with your fingers.

> Delicately open the outer lips and this time breathe (not blow) warm air on to the open vulva without touching it with your lips.

> Begin to explore the vulva with your fingers, moving very slowly and lightly from the outside inwards. Don't touch the clitoris yet. Read your partner's responses carefully and let them dictate your movement. Gradually build up rhythm and speed as if you were playing a living musical instrument.

> Use light flicking or rubbing movements, all the while using less pressure than you think they might be ready for so that their body movements continually beg you for more.

> When they are wet, dip your finger briefly into the vagina. Begin to explore it by darting in and out and let your partner thrust against you rather than press your fingers all the way in yourself. Keep withdrawing and playing with the vulva with your fingertips.

> Once you are deep inside the vagina, learn its shape, snugness and angle within the body. The better you know it, the more pleasure you can give during penetration.

• Fanny farts or 'queefs' are totally normal and can happen to anyone at any time.

! Never blow into the vagina – it could cause serious harm.

WATCH

You can learn a lot about how to touch your partner by watching them – male or female – masturbate. And then you can improve on their repertoire by adding imaginative variations of your own.

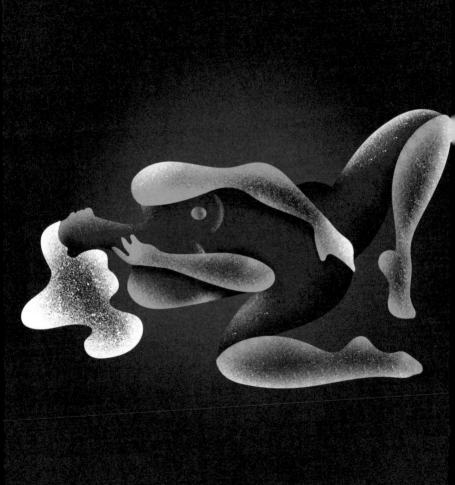

PERIOD PLAY

Yes it's messy but embrace the mess because it can also be also incredibly enjoyable. If mess is your biggest concern, lay some old towels down or get busy in the shower.

Some people report that period play can relieve cramps and headaches and intensify orgasms. Others find the smell and increased lubrication a real turn-on.

There's no medical reason most people can't play during menstruation (be mindful that it may not be for people with endometriosis) but you're still at risk of STIs and pregnancy is still possible so use the usual precautions.

The first 24–48 hours of some periods can be heavier and more painful and uncomfortable. If this is true for you, you may want to wait for the pain to ease.

Acupressure Points for Period Play

- **Meeting Point of the Three Yin Leg Meridians:** 3 *cun* (thumb's widths) above the tip of the ankle bone, push into the edge of the tibia. Especially useful when periods are irregular.
- **Heavenly Pivot:** 2 *cun* either side of the navel. Good for relieving menstrual pain.
- **Ocean of Blood:** 3 *cun* above the kneecap on the bulge of the muscle. As the name indicates, this is also good for menstrual pain.

THE PENIS AND TESTICLES

THE PENIS

The longest part of the penis is the shaft and the head or glans is at the tip of the shaft. The opening on the head is the urethra.

The hand-job technique

- Brush the flat of your palm along the insides of the legs, over the balls and quickly and lightly up the shaft, hardly touching the tip. Do this several times, increasing the pressure. The penis will strain up to meet your hand.
- Hold the shaft firmly in your hand and squeeze repeatedly, first very gently and then more firmly.
- Walk your fingers in small mischievous steps up the shaft and very lightly tickle the tip as it rises to meet you.
- If your partner is uncircumcised, hold the penis in your hand and make a snugly fitting circle with your forefinger and thumb just below the glans. Slowly pull the foreskin down. Stop. Squeeze. Raise the foreskin again. Take your time. Steadily build a rhythm. If they are circumcised, concentrate on the shaft, moving the foreskin up towards the glans then back down again.
- Make your movements confident, firm and leisurely. Give your partner the feeling you are totally in control and in no hurry.
- Towards the end, keep up the pressure and speed coolly and with control – your partner needs no distractions now – and when you feel their body tense in advance orgasm, hold on and carry through, not stopping until they subside.

More things to try

- Using two hands can increase the intensity. Encircle the base of the penis and grip it gently while using your other hand to stroke the shaft.
- Use lube or saliva to up the sensations. Don't be afraid to spit.
- Use twisting motions up and down the shaft and pull or tug gently.
- Play with their balls or slide your fingers underneath to gently knead the prostate.
- Tune in to their needs while you are masturbating them. Tantalize them by changing the rhythm or speed as well as by varying the angle and pressure you use.
- Try drumming your fingers on the shaft as if you were playing the flute.
- The underside of the glans can be incredibly sensitive, particularly the frenulum – the narrow strip of skin that connects the shaft with the head.

THE TESTICLES

In sex play, the testicles are often neglected, perhaps since everyone knows they are very pain-sensitive – but they also respond well to stimulation. Many adore having them caressed and licked.

> First, take a good look. They swell slightly with arousal, and move under the skin, creating an effect like waves out at sea. Just before ejaculation, they tighten and rise up under the penis.

> Pay attention to their inner thighs. Stroke them fleetingly with the palms of your hands, then push them apart and breathe hot air on them, barely touching them with your lips.

> Nuzzle the balls and trace the 'seam' between them with your tongue. Then playfully lick one then the other from below, working round the sides to the top.

> Pay attention to the perineum. Massage it with little walking steps with your fingers or tongue, pressing quite firmly, then swoop into feathery strokes all over the balls, alternating with cupping them in your hand and 'testing their weight'.

> With a firm tongue, lick vigorously and repeatedly from the upper corner of their thigh towards the point where penis and scrotum join. Then lick the testicle nearest to you with the same firm motion, occasionally 'accidentally' straying on to the root of the erect penis.

> After licking their testicles all over with little flicks, probing between them with the tip of your tongue to define their shape, nibble them with your lips, lick salaciously with the flat of your tongue, and gradually take one or both balls in your mouth. Use your lips and tongue only to manoeuvre them – keep your teeth covered by your lips.

- Some people like to have their balls gripped or cupped firmly and tugged slightly.

! The testicles can be extremely sensitive so check in with your partner regularly to ensure you're not causing them pain or discomfort.

THE P-SPOT

The prostate gland isn't technically included among the male genitalia but it's one of the most sensitive erogenous zones and sometimes referred to as the P-spot.

The prostate is a walnut-sized gland located under the perineum – between the scrotum and anus.

It can be reached internally through the anus – it's about 2 inches (5cm) inside on the front wall and feels a little like the tip of your nose. It can be stimulated by penetration – try massaging it with one finger pressing gently but firmly against it in a downward or circular stroking motion.

Or, massage the perineum with a thumb, knuckle or vibrator.

ORAL

The intimacy of mouth-to-genital contact is a powerful turn-on, both physically and emotionally. Physically, the super-sensitive tongue is a versatile instrument of pleasure for both sexes. From an emotional point of view, a certain level of intimacy, trust and lack of inhibition is required to surrender fully to the delights of oral sex.

IF THEY HAVE A CLITORIS (CUNNILINGUS)

More females experience an orgasm every time with oral sex than through any other form of sexual congress. This is because of the exquisite pleasure that the tongue can deliver by means of slippery, feathery or firm flicking movements over and around the clitoris. These tongue-generated orgasms are also generally more powerful than those given by the fingers.

Techniques to try

- Wait until your partner is fully aroused before making contact with the clitoris. The whole of the vulva will swell and flush, and the clitoris may well appear red and swollen from inside its hood.
- Get your partner to help you by communicating what feels best.
- Play 'the alphabet game' – writing capital letters with your tongue very slowly over your partner's open vulva, barely touching the clitoris as you pass.
- Probe into the vagina with your tongue, then try gentle firm pressure all over the vulva, letting your tongue 'dance'. A repeated light rhythmic flicking across the clitoris will usually have the effect of inducing the tension that releases into orgasm.
- With your partner's legs spread wide rest your head on one thigh and approach their clitoris from the side rather than above and flick your tongue quickly from side to side.
- Unless they encourage you otherwise, use the flat of your tongue rather than the tip as it can feel jabby to some.
- Parting their labia will fully expose their clitoris – if you want to finger them or explore their body with your hands, they can spread their labia.
- If they're lying down, place pillows under their hips so that their hips and vulva are thrust upwards.

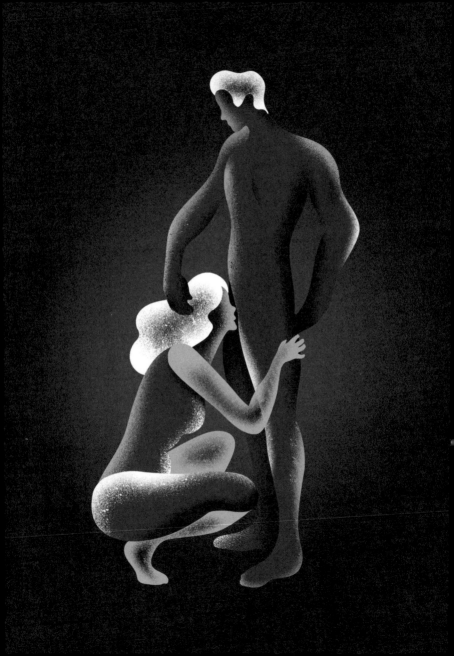

IF THEY HAVE A PENIS
(FELLATIO)

- Be prepared to move around your partner's body as you give them a blow job, so you can enjoy it from every angle.
- Nuzzle the shaft with the inside of your lips and apply pressure with the flat of your tongue as your mouth moves up and down towards the tip. Start at one side, move up and down the penis on top, then continue with the other side. Be energetic and thorough.
- Hold the penis in your hand and, lubricating it well, masturbate it slowly, lavishly licking and tickling the tip with your tongue. Keep up well-lubricated flowing movements, alternating all the time between hands and tongue, so your partner hardly knows where the sensation is coming from. Let your mouth follow your hand in a smooth rhythm.
- Curl your lips over your teeth and press your lips around their penis, or if they like it, gently graze your teeth up and down the shaft and gently over the tip.
- Now suck the tip of the penis and lubricate it with lots of saliva, moving your hand rapidly and lightly up and down the shaft, and tickling the opening of the urethra with the tip of your tongue.
- Feel your partner's whole body tense, then spasm as they come. Some may want you to carry on licking and sucking through several spasms, but with others, the glans becomes so sensitive that they can't bear contact any longer.
- If you are not going to swallow, try letting it squirt on to your lips and fingers and massaging it into the still throbbing penis until ejaculation stops and the movement subsides.

DEEP-THROAT

Deep-throat is exactly that – taking a penis deep into the back of your throat and although it can be pleasurable for both the giver and the receiver, it's not for everyone. How deeply the giver takes the penis into their mouth is down to them and sometimes it's going to boil down to physiology...some penises are too big and some mouths too small.

Power dynamics

Some people enjoy the kink of a submissive giver and dominant receiver. Here, the receiver is usually in control of their thrusts and the giver will gag and gasp for breath when they withdraw. Even if that's not something you want to try, deep-throat can be uncomfortable and trigger the gag reflex or make your eyes water so it's something to approach slowly.

- If you're the giver and want to avoid gagging completely, you'll need to breathe slowly and steadily through your nose.
- The giver must be able to control all movement.
- Every mouth is slightly different, as is every penis – some are straight, some curve, some heads are bigger than others...
- The angle of penetration will play a part in the giver's comfort so find a position that works for you. To begin, try it with the giver lying on a bed with their head off the edge and tilted.
- Some people are turned on by gagging noises so whether you're giving deep-throat or not, don't feel you need to keep the noise down.

ANAL PLAY

Anal play can be intensely pleasurable as the anus is a supersensitive area with lots of nerves. For some people the idea of anal play is a complete turn-off, so establish this well in advance.

RIMMING

Rimming refers to someone licking, kissing or probing their partner's anus with their tongue or fingers. It doesn't have to be penetrative – playing with the perineum and anal sphincter can be mind-blowing.

- Lick slowly upwards from the perineum across the anus with your tongue making broad strokes.
- Lick in circles around the opening with just the tip of your tongue.
- Kiss the anus with slow, soft kisses or trace your fingers gently across it.
- If you want to penetrate with your tongue, you don't need to go too deep. The first inch is the most sensitive so explore in slow circular movements with your tongue soft or clench your tongue and dart in and out.
- Experiment with speed and pressure.

PENETRATION

Anal penetration feels quite different to vaginal sex for the giver and the receiver. The anal sphincter clenches tightly onto the penis or toy.

For females, deep anal penetration can be the best way to stimulate the G-spot, which is located at the front wall of the vagina. If your partner is female, they could simultaneously insert a finger or toy into their vagina, or stimulate their clitoris.

The male prostate gland is the male G-spot and can be stimulated during anal penetration. It is located about 2 inches (5cm) inside the rectal passage towards the front of the body. Firm pressure applied here can lead to orgasm.

ANAL POSITIONS

If you're trying anal sex for the first time, these are the best positions to try.

- In **Doggy Style**, the receiver can reach around to grip the penis or toy to control how much of it enters the anus.
- In **Cow Girl**, the penetrator brings their knees up to support the receiver's weight slightly while the receiver can bring themselves gently onto the penis or toy and is able to control entry.
- From **Missionary**, the receiver can twist slightly so that both ankles are on the penetrator's shoulders.

Tips to try

- If you want to try it, make sure you're fully aroused and completely relaxed before you begin.
- Before moving on to sex, gently massage or rim your partner's anus without penetration. Then begin penetration – start slowly and don't go too deep. Some like a finger to slide in and out or a finger to swivel and rotate.
- Lubricate the penis, strap-on or toy well and proceed gently, at first just entering the anus with the tip and resting there a while, then working with and not against the muscles of the anus as they gradually allow you in. Let your partner dictate how deeply and strongly you thrust.
- The receiver should be pushing out with the anal muscles rather than holding them tight, or it could hurt.

! Anal sex can be painful for the beginner receiver. If you feel pain, stop and apply more lube or spend time on other forms of play to get you more aroused. If it's still painful, stop. You could try experimenting with an anal training kit – a set of butt plugs of various sizes – that can get you used to and more comfortable with being penetrated. Start small and work your way up.

! Some people (givers and receivers) get the ick about traces of poo but let's step back here and consider the anus and rectum's primary function. If you're not down with the natural, play elsewhere. Although douching is a popular and oft-touted method of 'cleaning up' before anal play, it's rarely necessary and done too much, can cause harm.

PEGGING

Pegging refers (usually) to a partner with a penis receiving anal penetration with a strap-on worn by someone without a penis.

Pegging stimulates the prostate gland but beyond the physical side of pleasure, pegging can bring a fun new dynamic to sex. Reversing the traditional giver and receiver roles can be empowering and also downright arousing.

Pegging often feels strange at first to people with vaginas as the hips can instinctively want to stir or rotate. Focus on thrusting as much as possible – arch your back and then clench your buttocks as you thrust forward.

❗ Because the rectum lining is thinner and more easily damaged than the vaginal wall, STIs are more easily transmitted via anal sex than vaginal sex. Fingernails can also snag the membrane and transmit infection. Be scrupulous with hygiene and always use a condom or a latex glove.

❗ Don't penetrate the vagina after the anus without washing thoroughly, or you could transfer bacteria from one to the other. Also take care if inserting a sex toy into the anus – the rectal passage can suck objects inside itself. Make sure your dildo is flared at the bottom, with no rough edges.

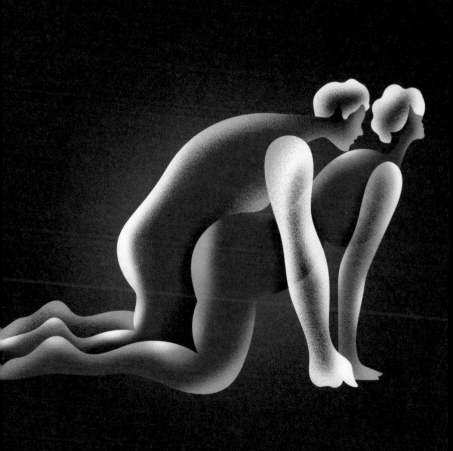

FISTING

Fisting isn't just 'a porn thing' – it's very much a real world thing, too. Some people love the sense of fullness that fisting gives, and like to explore how much they can fit inside them. Fisting can lead to incredibly intense orgasms.

It's really important to go slow, and before trying fisting for the first time, it's a good idea to incorporate toys into your sex play. Start small and slowly build up to bigger and bigger dildos.

BEFORE YOU TRY

- Spend a lot of time on getting your partner aroused first so that they're relaxed.
- You will need a LOT of lube.
- Trim the fingernails right down and buff them to avoid scratching.
- Remove any rings or jewellery.
- ! Never splay the fingers wide once inside and don't make sudden movements. If the receiver feels any pain. Stop immediately.

HOW TO DO IT

The name fisting is misleading – you aren't making a fist and inserting it into a vagina or anus. You're actually making a conical shape (like an elongated goose head) with your fingers by bringing them together. First and third fingers tucked under the middle finger, pinky finger tucked under those, thumb tucked right in under the fingers between the palm and first joint of the fingers. The closer the thumb is to the tip of your fingers, the more of a right angle shape you'll create – this is often too big if you're new to fisting so keep it tucked low.

- Initially, insert only the tips of 3 fingers and move in slow, stirring motions.
- Keep applying lube and gently push the fingers further and further in.

DOUBLE PENETRATION

Double penetration (DP) usually refers to both the anus and vagina being penetrated simultaneously. 'Spit roasting' is commonly used to refer to the anus OR vagina AND the mouth being penetrated but with so many variations on the theme, it's easier to think of DP as referring to any two orifices being penetrated at the same time.

It's also possible for multiple toys, fingers or penises to be inserted in a single orifice simultaneously, while something else penetrates another so you'll also hear of triple and quadruple penetration.

You can explore double penetration through solo masturbation using fingers or toys before involving a partner or partners.

! Always use plenty of lube and if there's a penis and a toy involved pay extra attention to what types of lube you're using. Remember that silicone toys will be damaged by silicone lube.

! If you have a vagina, ensure that nothing inserted into your anus is inserted into your vagina without a change of condom or thorough wash.

! If you're playing with others and are inserting anything into your mouth – be it a toy, penis or ball gag – establish safe words or gestures in advance.

DEEPER PENETRATION

Deeper penetration literally hits the spots further back
in both the vagina and rectum.

- Use pillows or cushions to augment positions. In
  Missionary, place a pillow under the receiver's
  buttocks to lift their pelvis higher. If the receiver is
  lying face down, place pillows under their chest so that
  their back arches and pushes their hips outwards; or
  place pillows under their hips to lift them.
- If your partner is lying down with you straddling them,
  bring your feet on to their chest if you are facing one
  another, or if you're straddling them in reverse, bring
  your feet together inside their legs, as close to their
  groin as possible.
- In Missionary, the receiver spreads their legs wide,
  grips their ankles and brings them back as close to
  their head as possible – this requires some flexibility
  and don't attempt this if you suffer from low back pain
  or hip issues.
- In Cow Girl, the penetrator grips their partner's hips
  and lifts them as they push up and pulls them back
  down as they lower themselves.

! It should never be painful so go slowly and if you suffer
  from endometriosis, bowel issues or anything else that
  may be likely to cause pain, be extremely cautious and
  stop immediately if you experience pain.

PLAYING WITH
THE SENSES

Although sight and touch are most associated with sex, all five senses – touch, sight, hearing, smell and taste – combine during play and stimulating every one simultaneously is the key to the most satisfying sex. But equally, denying one of the senses can heighten the others.

SOUND

As mentioned, the ears are an erogenous zone.

- **Moan, whisper** or simply **breathe** into your partner's ear during sex.
- **Express yourself** and don't hold back your natural voiced response to sex – it's yet another inhibition to relinquish. It's often a boost to your partner's libido to hear that you're enjoying yourself, too.
- **Talk dirty**. If you feel self-conscious talking, blindfold your partner.
- If you're not ready to explore your vocal side, or find silence distracting, introduce **music** to sex sessions and create a 'sex mix' to set the tone.

SIGHT

- **Watching your partner** is a turn-on and increases intimacy and trust. Make eye contact as you massage, lick or suck each other's bodies.
- **Mirrors**. Play in front of a full-length mirror. While that idea is scary to some, it's a proven way to build self-confidence and helps you find your inner exhibitionist. Visual stimulation is, like touch, a turn-on and seeing yourself during sex will both arouse you further, and show you just how strong, sensuous or beautiful you are. Mirror sex gives you an all-new perspective of your and your partner's bodies – face the mirror while taking it from behind and make eye contact. Or turn to watch each other in the mirror.

LIGHTS ON OR OFF?

Do you like to play with the lights on or off, or somewhere in between? If you feel self-conscious in anything other than the dark, it's time to explore what's going on emotionally. Good, healthy sex relies on mutual trust and appreciation. Get to know and love your own body and discard any notions of ideal or normal body types. There is no such thing.

You should always feel comfortable, so pay attention to lighting, and discuss your worries with your partner. If you feel self-conscious in bright light but want the intimacy of being able to see your partner, create pools of soft light away from the bed so that you can see enough to read each other's eyes. Try candles, or fit dusky pink, red or even black light bulbs into a lamp.

BLINDFOLDS

Denying your partner sight will increase their sensitivity to touch. In longer-term sexual relationships, a switch to sex with an element of anonymity can give an extra frisson of danger and help to strip away inhibitions you never knew you had. Explore one another's body by touch alone, or guide them by voice.

- Keep it slow and full of surprises. Experiment with different sensations – texture, temperature, pressure – on various parts of their body. Graze their skin with your nipples or genitals.
- Find out which parts are most sensitive to each mystery stimulant – get them to guess what's happening to them.

SMELL

'Love chemicals', or pheromones, are chemicals that animals use to communicate and, particularly in the animal kingdom, play a part in attracting a mate. Pheromones are found in our bodily fluids including vaginal fluids, semen, sweat, urine and breastmilk and may help us in attracting a mate.

But it isn't just pheromones that are at play during sex. Our bodily odours are incredibly attractive to sexual partners and unless your own are objectively foul (which would be unusual) or stale, don't be in a rush to seek to mask them. Although everyone's scent will be different, most can be described as musky, slightly sour, slightly sweet or even animal. If you do want to play with scent, experiment with essential oils, lotions or juices with fragrances known for their aphrodisiac or performance-enhancing properties.

- **Jasmine**, **Ylang Ylang** and **Vanilla**, **Strawberry** and **Cinnamon** are all lauded for their aphrodisiac effects.
- **Ylang Ylang**, **Sandalwood**, **Lavender** and **Clary Sage** may contribute to a higher state of female arousal and more intense orgasm.
- **Ginseng**, **Rose**, **Lavender** and **Clove** may boost male libido, increase blood flow and circulation within the penis and counter erectile dysfunction.

TASTE

We'll talk more about taste in SEX AND FOOD but it's worth talking about the all-natural side of bodies and taste. As with smell, don't hurry to disguise your body's secretions.

- **Vaginal fluids** – and the labia, and vulva – can taste sweet, salty, slightly sour or slightly sharp and the taste may change throughout the menstrual cycle or with increased levels of sweat. All of these tastes are healthy, natural and normal – vaginas don't naturally smell of roses.
- **Semen** often tastes slightly salty or metallic with a freshness resembling cucumber or mild chlorine.
- A clean **anus**, as well as fluids and secretions within a clean rectum, will smell 'warm' and slightly musky. But no matter what steps you take to clean yourself, there is always the chance of the rectum smelling of (or containing traces of) faeces and that is only ever normal. If either you or your partner isn't reassured by this, anal play might not be for you.
- There's anecdotal evidence to suggest that foods such as pineapple, mango and asparagus can make both semen and vaginal fluids taste sweeter, and that spices such as cumin, turmeric and garlic can alter the taste.

SEX AND FOOD

The body's most important sex organ is the brain – and when it comes to aphrodisiacs you can be sure it's almost always in the mind.

- Food can be a powerful aphrodisiac, so serve it in the most sensual way you can imagine.
- Feed each other with your lips and drink from each other's skin. The way you eat can hold the promise of what you will do to your partner with your mouth and fingers later.
- **Dark chocolate** stimulates the brain to produce serotonin and phenylethylamine. Phenylethylamine is a hormone-like substance that produces that euphoric, dizzying sensation we get when we fall in love, and serotonin is the social chemical that boosts our mood, confidence and self-esteem.
- **Nakedness** tends to go very well with foods that **drizzle**, **squash**, **wobble** or **melt**. Try **chocolate sauce**, **mousse**, **ice cream**, **honey**, **molasses** or **strawberries**. Chocolate and honey particularly arouse all five senses and prime your body for sex. Smear them over your nipples, toes, earlobes or behind your knees; or drizzle them into your navel, over your testicles or along your inner thigh.
- **!** Sugar can trigger yeast infections so avoid contact with the vagina, inner labia, glans or opening to the urethra.

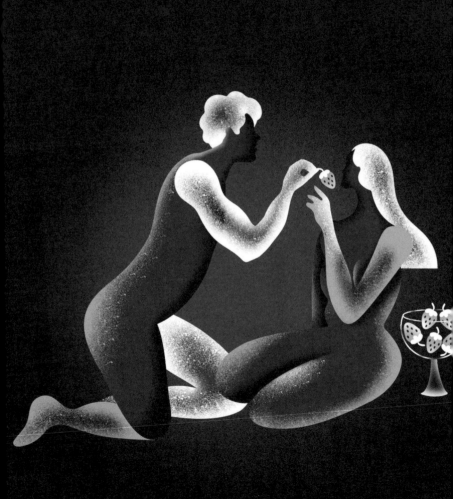

FOOD PLAY

- *Nyotaimori* is probably one of the best known forms of food play. It's the act of serving sushi or sashimi on a female body. *Nantaimori* is the male equivalent. If sushi isn't your thing, use your favourite foods. Stipulate that the food must be eaten without using the fingers – only lips and tongue allowed!

- Vegetables such as **cucumber**, **maize** and **root vegetables**, or fruits such as bananas are a tempting substitute for sex toys but as with sugar, they can trigger infections and affect the vagina's pH. If food insertion is something you want to try, always use condoms.

- For added kink, try **figging**. Figging is the act of inserting a piece of peeled, raw ginger into the anus or vagina. It causes a tingling, burning sensation which can drive some people wild.

- ! If you're anal figging, carve the ginger into the shape of a butt plug to avoid it getting lost in there.

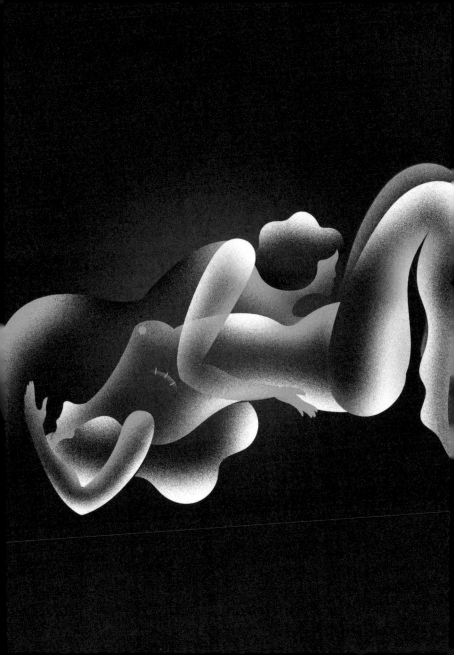

ORGASMS

First up, you do not have to orgasm or come during sex to enjoy sex. Sex play can be, and is, pleasurable without orgasm.

There's nuance here, and you have to focus first on what sex means to you, and your partner. The pressure to 'perform' or show 'ultimate satiation' is an artificial construct. Many of us are taught that sex is a biological act designed only to make babies and it isn't about pleasure. Huh, so why the female orgasm? Why the pleasure from anal sex? Why deny yourself the pleasure of riding a dildo?

Sometimes, no matter how much we're aroused, we just can't or don't orgasm. You haven't failed and you haven't let anyone down. If you don't orgasm but that's OK with you, that's OK. If your partner doesn't orgasm but that's OK with them, that's OK, too.

But if you want to orgasm, or you want to make your partner orgasm, here are some tips...

MAKING IT LAST

TANTRIC BLISS AND EDGING

The art of tantric sex can take years to perfect – but you can introduce some tantric techniques into your sex life to add variety, intensify orgasms and help sex last longer.

Tantric sex is really all about techniques that establish the ultimate mind-body connection. It's about slowing sex down and enjoying it for longer, and not just focus on the orgasm. Think of it as 'mindful' sex.

Experts use yoga and meditation but for a beginner, **the key points to remember are to take your time, pause before you reach the peak and maintain eye contact with your partner** – something that's probably much more difficult than you think.

Edging is the act of barrelling towards orgasm only to stop, cease all stimulation so that the sensation subsides and then start the build-up again.

TANTRIC TIPS FOR SLOWING DOWN PENETRATIVE SEX

- Use lots of lubricant to create less friction, because friction is what stimulates you.
- Start by sitting on the floor with your partner sitting astride you in your lap. Instead of them bouncing up and down, just hold one another, occasionally rocking back and forth. Gaze into each other's left eye... What happens? See how long you can keep this up.
- Avoid building up a thundering rhythm. Vary your thrusts or bounces between slow and deep and quick and shallow.
- Stop thrusting, rocking or grinding. Stay still, hold the pose and take deep, regular breaths, breathing from your belly not your chest. Concentrate on your breathing until the urgency has passed.
- Stay completely still, relax the genital and anal muscles and press your tongue against the roof of your mouth behind your teeth. Concentrate on the contact your tongue is making until the feeling of approaching climax subsides.
- Variety is the key – make a change every time you feel yourself about to lose control.
- The stop-start technique involves just that – every time you reach a peak of excitement and feel yourself about to let go, stop and, not withdrawing, stay very still inside your partner until you feel the urgency pass and can begin to move again.

IF YOU HAVE A PENIS

- As you get nearer to orgasm, the testicles rise up tightly under the penis. To slow down, stop thrusting, stay still and gently hold your testicles down using the palm of one hand – or get your partner to do this for you. Wait a while before you begin again.
- Avoid pulling out so much that you stimulate the head of the penis as you drive back in again. Then combine the two – try going in slow, low and deep and coming out fast, pulling your body upwards as you do so. With you on top this stimulates the sensitive front of the vagina or rectum.
- Withdraw your penis a little, so that only the glans remains inside the vagina or anus. Hold the position until the urgency has passed, then slowly enter again.
- If you're getting too excited, withdraw and give your partner oral sex. Don't worry about going limp for a while, your partner's increased arousal will soon get you going again.

BREATHE

Orgasms can be intensified by breath work. In the minute before orgasm, slow the breathing down so that each inhale and exhale lasts 4–5 seconds. As the breathing slows, tighten the PC muscles.

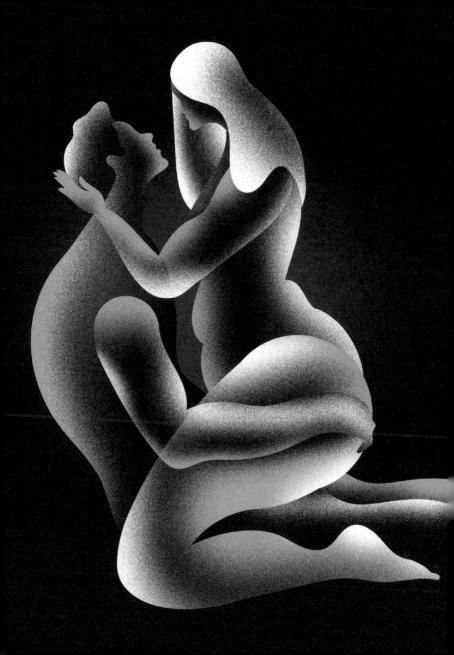

SPEEDING UP

- Being on top is a good way to encourage an orgasm as it gives you the opportunity to set the pace. Face the toes to feel the pressure of the penis on the front wall of the vagina or rectum and get deep penetration.
- Try a receiver-on-top position: face your partner's head and lie on their chest. You will need to be very vigorous as you drag your body upwards. Clench the vaginal or anal muscles and really tug at your partner's penis or toy as if you were using your hand. Grind back down in a circular motion, then drag up again – exquisite for both of you.

COMING TOGETHER

Some people claim that simultaneous orgasm is the best thing that ever happened to them, while others find it a bit bewildering – the pleasure of your partner's orgasm is lost behind the explosion of your own, leaving you wondering what happened. You're not missing anything if it doesn't happen to you, but you can have a lot of fun experimenting with timing. It will add to your knowledge of each other's sexual responses and help make sex last longer.

TIPS FOR FEMALE ORGASMS

In relationships in which a male and a female is involved, some of the difficulty in getting the timing right lies in the fact that the female orgasm tends to be a slower and more complex sexual response than the male orgasm.

Although all orgasms are equal, people with vaginas and clitorises do report different sensations according to whether they are being penetrated or masturbated. Masturbatory orgasms, which are experienced by all people who can teach themselves to come through masturbation, alone or with a partner, are the more pleasurably acute. All those who orgasm in this way know the acute tension of the clitoris, the voluptuous rushing sensation that breaks into multiple contractions of the surrounding tissue.

A small minority of females (around 20 per cent, according to sex researcher Shere Hite), who also orgasm with a penis inside the vagina, describe that as a quite different experience. Although Freud claimed that orgasms experienced during intercourse were superior to those without intercourse, the majority of females in a survey carried out by Shere Hite said they were less intense. Whereas masturbatory orgasm is experienced as a high, sweet, rippling sensation, the peak of sensitivity, orgasm with penetration is like the boom of a distant explosion, powerful, but somewhat muffled.

Orgasms triggered by the partner's fingers or tongue, and by masturbation, are probably more intense because stimulation is more localized and more sensitively guided.

Orgasm during penetration is undoubtedly quite rare for many females because a thrusting penis can stimulate the clitoris only 'in passing', if at all, depending on the position of the couple. The orgasm experienced during intercourse may be more diffuse because the penis or toy alters the focus of attention from the clitoris alone to the whole of the lower part of the body, and because the vagina is full, the sensation becomes rather 'muffled'.

- Sit on your partner's lap facing away from them. While rocking tightly back and forwards, your partner holds your labia open with one hand and fondles around your clitoris with the fingers of the other, giving you a stretched-to-bursting feeling that you wouldn't get if they actually touched your clitoris.

CLITORAL STIMULATION

Some penetrative positions stimulate the clitoris and labia without the need for fingers or vibrators.

- The penetrating partner sits on the side of the bed with the receiver straddling them, with either feet or knees on the bed. This allows the receiver to push and rub against the penetrator as they rock or bounce.
- In Cow Girl, rock to and fro instead of bouncing or pushing up with your legs. Rock slowly and grind hard against their body.
- In many positions, the penetrating partner can 'stir' or rotate their hips rather than thrust.
- Many people find the clitoris is too sensitive to touch after they come. Ask what they like – often this is the best time for penetration.

SQUIRTING AND FEMALE EJACULATION

'Squirting' has trickled (well, gushed) into mainstream conversation via porn but there's a load of confusion about what it is and whether it's something anyone can do.

First up, squirting is not female ejaculation despite the two terms often being used interchangeably.

Female ejaculation refers to the slightly thick, milky white liquid that accompanies orgasms in some females. The quantity of this liquid varies from person to person but it's rarely enough to soak a sheet.

Squirting, on the other hand, refers to the sudden expulsion of a more significant amount of liquid that's usually clear and thin. Despite countless studies, scientists can't quite agree on what this liquid is so if all you want to know is 'is it pee, or not?', we can't help. There's usually urine present in the fluid, and it definitely comes from the bladder, but the chemical make-up is very different to urine. And no, it doesn't smell or taste of urine.

Squirting isn't necessarily linked to orgasm but is only triggered by intense arousal. Some people will squirt without an orgasm – and sometimes multiple times – and some people will squirt as they orgasm. As to whether it's something anyone with a vagina and vulva can do, the jury's out. Some people hold the problematic line that anyone can squirt 'if their partner knows what they're doing', while in the real world, many others have partners who know exactly what they're doing but have never squirted.

TRY IT

Squirting is not the gold standard of female arousal and as with most things, trying to do something just for the sake of doing it is unlikely to be enjoyable. If you want to try it, put pleasure first – it's all about the intense stimulation of the G-spot, and is helped along by clitoral stimulation.

- When they are fully aroused, have your partner sit on the edge of the bed, legs splayed and feet and bum on the bed. They should lean back slightly or lie back. Comfort is key here.
- Using two fingers or a toy (a G-spot wand would be perfect) begin to stimulate the G-spot – gently at first and then applying more pressure and building a rhythm. Some people enjoy a sustained and very vigorous rhythm and find that it is more likely to trigger squirting.
- Suck on their clitoris or massage it with your other hand as you continue to work on the G-spot.
- Many people report that they feel a sudden need to 'pee' just before squirting and the giver can usually tell that their partner is reaching the peak of pleasure. At this point withdraw the toy or fingers quickly, or move them down and away from the front wall of the vagina so that the tubes aren't compressed and the fluid can squirt out.

CERVICAL ORGASMS

Some females can have cervical orgasms and report them to be more intense than clitoral or labial orgasms.

- The cervix is the protruding fleshy nub at the back of the vagina. Its position and the way it feels will change with arousal as well as throughout the menstrual cycle. Sometimes, it will feel soft, open and closer to the vaginal opening while at other times it will harden, close and retract further back.
- The cervix can be very sensitive, and some people will find any contact at all with the cervix causes discomfort or pain so it is always best explored first by its owner!
- Sometimes, your own fingers will reach the cervix but it's often more comfortable to use a long, slim toy to probe around its edges and press against it. You can press with as much pressure as feels right – the opening is tiny and you needn't worry about penetrating it.
- Sweep around and around in circular motions, pausing to stop and push against its sides. Flick the toy up and over the cervix or make pulsing movements across the opening.

OVER AND OVER

Multiple and sequential orgasms, like vaginal and
clitoral orgasms, are concepts that have caused
a lot of confusion and left many people worried
that their sexual response might be inadequate.
Never worry about that.

Because orgasms come in waves, some people are not
even sure whether their orgasms are multiple or single.
Multiple orgasms are those that are experienced in a
chain, one directly after another; sequential orgasms
are those with a gap of a few minutes between each one.
It seems that true multiple orgasm is extremely rare,
although many women are capable of sequential orgasm.

Being capable of six orgasms in a row is not the same
as needing or even wanting that many. According to
Shere Hite, about 90 per cent of people who orgasm feel
completely satisfied with a single climax. And in many
people the clitoris remains hypersensitive, and further
stimulation is uncomfortable and can even prove painful.

PREMATURE EJACULATION

Premature ejaculation is very common and can be caused by trauma, stress, anxiety, erectile dysfunction, genetic and health problems, difficulties within relationships and everything in between. Alcohol and drugs can also exacerbate premature ejaculation.

As with everything else, communication, and ensuring your partner is comfortable at all times, is key. Premature ejaculation should never be (but inevitably often is) a cause of shame, fear or embarrassment.

Several techniques can help males last longer and delay ejaculation, but these should be used in conjunction with examining the cause of the problem. Understanding what is wrong often brings its own release. For example, a fear of intimacy may contribute to premature ejaculation. Intimacy always brings with it the risk of loss, and the unbearable pain attendant on that loss. Subconsciously, a male who gets sex over and done with quickly may be trying to protect himself from close emotional involvement.

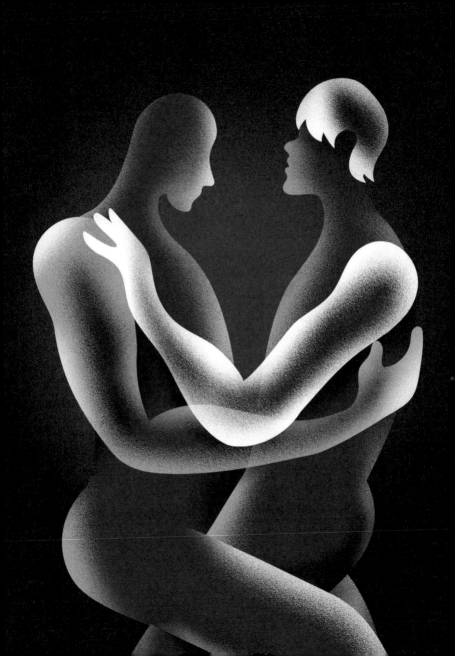

THE STOP-START TECHNIQUE
FOR DELAYING EJACULATION

The aim of these exercises is to learn to keep yourself below the point at which ejaculation seems inevitable for as long as possible.

Tips for when you're on your own

These tips can help you gain and build a sense of self-control:

> **Step one** Masturbate with a dry hand. Avoid fantasizing, and concentrate instead on the sensation in your penis. Allow the pleasure to build up but stop immediately when you feel you are about to lose control. Relax for a while, still keeping your mind free of fantasies, until the chance of ejaculation has passed, then begin again. Following the same pattern, aim to continue stopping and starting for 15 minutes without orgasm. You may not be able to manage it at first, but keep trying. As you get more practised, you will probably find you have to stop less often. When you have completed three 15-minute sessions on three consecutive occasions proceed to step two.

> **Step two** involves masturbating with lubrication to heighten sensation, and make delay more difficult. Follow step one until you have completed three separate consecutive sessions.

> **Step three** You will now have gained a good measure of control. Now masturbate with a dry hand for 15 minutes before ejaculation. Keep focusing on your penis rather than fantasizing. When you feel yourself getting dangerously excited, don't stop, but instead, change rhythm or alter your strokes in such a way that the pressure to ejaculate fades. Experiment to see which strokes excite you most, and which allow you most control. Work on this step until you have completed three consecutive sessions.

Now involve your partner

> **Step four** Lie on your back and get them to masturbate you with a dry hand, as in step one. Concentrate on the sensations in your penis and ask them to stop every time you get too aroused before the time is up. Aim to last for three consecutive 15-minute sessions.

> **Step five** Repeat step four, but your partner should use a lubricant while they masturbate you. You will find ejaculation much more difficult to control, and you may have to ask them to stop more often. Once you have mastered three consecutive 15-minute sessions, you are ready to try the stop-start technique with intercourse.

> **Step six** The best position for delaying ejaculation is with your partner on top. Once you are inside them, ask them to move gently. Put your hands on their hips so that you can let them know with your hands when you want them to stop, and when you are ready for them to start again. Again, aim to last for 15 minutes, but if you can't, don't worry; you can start again once you recover your erection, and the second time

you will probably have more control. During intercourse, concentrate entirely on yourself. Give your partner your full concentration and bring them to orgasm before or afterwards, with oral or manual stimulation.

THE SQUEEZE TECHNIQUE FOR DELAYING EJACULATION

The 'squeeze' action is designed to cause your erection to subside, and it can be applied every time you get too close to ejaculation.

> Your partner performs the squeeze by gripping your penis firmly, and pressing with their thumb on the frenulum. This is the place on the underside of the penis where the head joins the shaft. At the same time, they press on the opposite side of the penis with their forefinger, and with their other fingers curled round the shaft.

• It is important that they press fairly hard on the penis and don't move their hand while doing so. Too light a touch could cause you to ejaculate straight away.

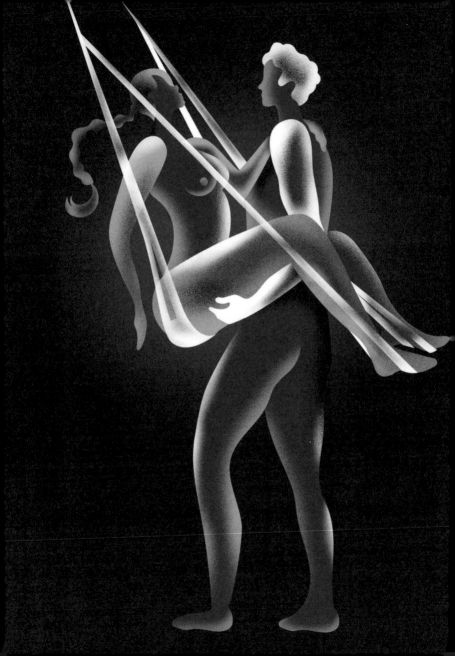

VARIETY

Playing erotic games together puts the all-too-often-missing element of fun back into your sex life. Role-playing, sharing and enacting your fantasies and using toys to excite one another can all add new dimensions. Planning ahead increases the anticipation and excitement. Every now and again, make a date with your partner and devote it to trying something new. Take it in turns to choose what will be on the menu. The preparation should all be part of the fun.

BEYOND THE BEDROOM

The desire for sex any time and anywhere ensures a level of adventurousness and spontaneity. Not all of us have that desire, or it is inhibited by worries or a lack of inspiration, and for some of us it can disappear as relationships develop. To make things fun and keep things fresh, take your play out of the bedroom and into the bathroom, outdoors and even, secretly, into public places.

Something about sex in the open is truly erotic – nowhere else will you feel so naked, so spontaneous, or so natural. Sex outside connects with the rhythms of nature, bringing an exquisite vulnerability. The possibility of discovery by others is part of the thrill. Remember though, if you are caught, you could be charged with sexual offences so the advice would be to only ever have sex outside when and where there is a reasonable expectation of privacy!

WATER PLAY

The bathroom provides a natural environment for sex and is also a favourite place for masturbation. The heat of the water increases blood flow and the jets of water stimulate nerve endings across the body.

THINGS TO DO IN THE SHOWER

- **Watch your partner** masturbate. Sit mesmerized in a chair while they put on a show for you in the shower. Watch as they come.
- **Water massage** With the temperature just right and the shower on full, give your partner a water massage. A shower head is great for massaging – some love it so much that they come as the water gently needles their vulva and clitoris or their testicles.
- **Lathering up** Use plenty of soap or shower gel to make each other hot and slippery.
- **!** Don't be tempted to use soap or gel as a lube as it can cause irritation and infection. And it burns.

- **Golden showers** Perhaps the idea of urinating on one another is too kink for some but the shower is the best place to experiment. If it's new to you and you're unsure, the water will wash it all away immediately. If it works for you, turn the shower off when you start to flow, so you can feel the warmth of each other's urine.

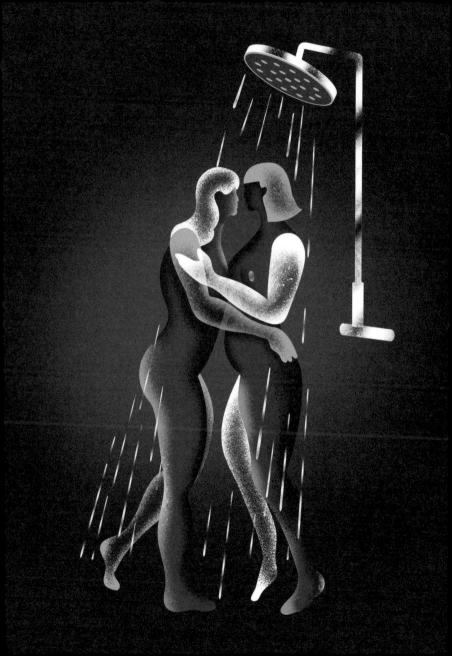

THINGS TO DO IN THE BATH.

- Make bathtime something special by sharing it. In the evening, add candles, music, oils or rose petals sprinkled on the water. Or suggest having a bath in the middle of the day as a surprise to completely lift your mood, particularly if it is cold and wet outside. Add masses of foam.
- Give your partner an underwater massage. Pay special attention to areas of tension around the neck and shoulders first, so they are completely relaxed before you start to massage the genitals. Use gently probing fingers to explore your partner's pelvic area. This can move to mutual masturbation when you're ready.
- When you're ready for sex, the size of your bath is going to determine which positions to try – in a small tub, try seated and reverse seated positions.
- Take toys into the bath with you to make bathtime more playful.
- The bath is the perfect place to experiment with penetrating your partner's vagina or anus with your toes.
- Combine bath time with a steamy mutual grooming session – wash and perhaps pull the hair if that's your partner's thing, shave each other, or pay special attention to the feet.
- Water, paradoxically, is drying. Apply plenty of lube before you immerse yourselves.

FAST AND FURIOUS

When anticipation is high and there's no scope for any prolonged play – at parties, in the park, on the beach – you'll need to get creative with penetrative positions and work at a pace that will get you over the line before you're caught. And that's all part of the fun. Angles of deep penetration are good for fast, furious sex.

POSITIONS FOR FAST SEX

- The penetrating partner sits (on toilets, stairs, rocks) and the receiver straddles them, arms around their necks. Or, reverse the straddle so that the receiver is facing away. This is a position of deep penetration. The partner who is sat down can help by holding their partner firmly at the waist and thrusting upwards as they bounce.
- Bend over anything – a sink, a chair or bench – while the penetrating partner stands and enters them from behind. The higher the receiver's hips are, and the more the back is arched, the deeper the penetration.
- In tight spaces, use carrying positions. Stand on the toilet in front of your penetrating partner who is also stood up. Have your partner clasp their hands behind your back and lower yourself down onto them with your arms around their neck. The penetrating partner can lean back against a wall for support so that your weight is on them, or if they're strong enough to do so, can lean you against the wall and thrust into you.

PLAYTIME

Adult forays into new sexual territory can mask
hungry curiosity with riotous silliness – it shoos away
the threat of taboo. Introducing games into your sex
life can inject a sense of fun and spontaneity. There
are hundreds of sexy twists on classic card and board
games available, or for easy DIY ideas, try these...

FUN GAMES TO PLAY

- **Forfeits** Saucy forfeits can be incorporated into any
  existing board game or card game. Have two sets of
  cards – one with actions, such as touch, tickle, kiss,
  suck, and another with body parts. The player has to
  apply the action to the correct body part.
- **Confessional forfeits** The forfeit cards have
  incomplete sentences on them, such as 'The first
  time I touched a naked person...'. The player has to
  complete the sentence.
- **Darts** Write filthy suggestions on pieces of paper
  pinned to a dart board. Then take it in turns to throw
  darts, and do whatever the speared pieces of paper tell
  you to.
- **Charades** Each team gives the other the title of an
  erotic book or film to enact without words. Imaginary
  titles are just as good as, if not better than, real ones.
- **When the music stops** Play an adult version of this
  game, involving stripping or sexual favours.

FANTASY

ROLE PLAY

It's easy to let the pressure to do it right make us forget that sex is all about playing together. So, what sexy games do you play in your daydreams? Lots of people have fantasies about their current partners that involve a surprising shift.

Role play is a great way to explore sharing fantasies and if you're embarrassed to share your own with your partner initially, there are some fun, stock roles to try.

- **Fancy dress** Go where the imagination takes you – the drama and erotic mystery of a masked ball has always offered the opportunity for the sexual alter ego to run amok.
- **Doctors and nurses** Playing at being sexologists. The sexologist is there to study the patient's sexual response in depth – so anything goes...
- **Customs officer and smuggler** This involves a uniform, a full-body search, smuggled goods and bribery with sexual favours...
- **Caught unawares** You think you're alone, and embark on some abandoned self-gratification. However, a voyeur is so enjoying your every move that they give themselves away. Far from being angry or embarrassed, you invite them to join in.

FANTASIES AND RELATIONSHIPS

Fantasies are worth sharing – and swapping one of yours for one of your partner's – and acting them out could make your sex life take off like a rocket. But, particularly if you're in a committed relationship, be careful about revealing fantasies that involve a third person – your partner may not be so keen to hear that you fantasize about their best friend or parent. Of course, it's understood that having a fantasy about someone doesn't mean you're looking for an opportunity to play with them in real life, but be mindful of your partner's emotions and how you communicate with one another.

TOY BOX

GOOD VIBRATIONS

Dildos – even double dildos that could be used by two
women – have been known since Stone Age times.

The first electrical dildos, or vibrators, were produced in
America around 1910. They were large, cumbersome machines
designed to be used by doctors on female patients suffering
from hysteria – 'womb disease' – what we today would call
sexual frustration. But it wasn't until the feminist revolution
of the 1960s and 70s when females were able to talk openly
about pleasure (and be heard!) and the fact that orgasm is not
always easily achieved through penetration, that vibrators (or
vibrating dildos) started to be marketed as a sexual device.

Today there are hundreds of toys available for everyone
regardless of gender – vibrating or otherwise. Single or
double; with or without ears to stimulate the A-spot, G-spot
or clitoris; wands, eggs, beads, balls, sleeves, rings – if you can
imagine it, someone has probably made it.

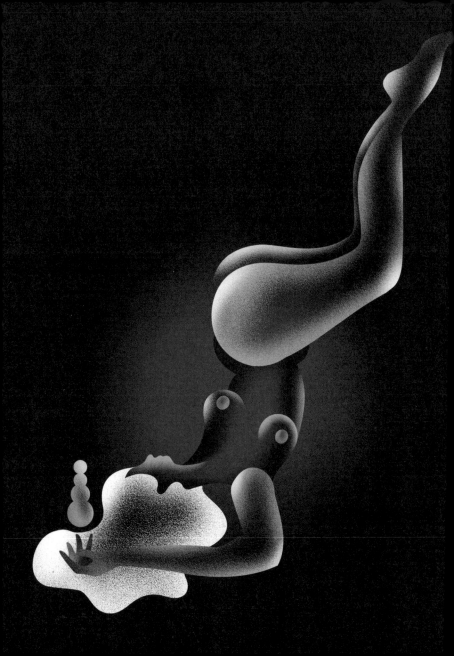

- The terms '**dildo**' and '**vibrator**' are sometimes used interchangeably but they're two different things. Dildos are usually phallus, hand or tentacle shaped and intended for insertion, and don't necessarily vibrate. They come in a variety of sizes and can enhance all kinds of play. Some have a suction cup at the base which allows you to mount them on a wall or mirror, others are double-ended for mutual pleasure.
- **Wands** and **vibrators** can be phallus shaped and vibrate, squirm or rotate. Some are designed for insertion while others are designed for external stimulation. There are a host of smaller, discrete vibrators that are remote controlled for hands-free fun.
- **Balls and eggs** are designed to be inserted into the vagina. Part toner, part toy, they literally 'jiggle', encouraging the muscles to contract to keep them in place. They can be worn for hours to strengthen muscles, or inserted just before sex to stimulate lubrication and blood flow.
- **Beads** are a series of balls on a 'string' with a grip at one end. They are inserted into the vagina or rectum – slowly for maximum pleasure – and then removed quickly or slowly before or during orgasm.
- **Butt plugs** are similar to dildos but tend to be tapered and have a flared end to prevent them getting lost.
- **Masturbators** are devices that fit over the penis. They have openings designed to look like a vagina or anus (or ankle for the foot fetishists) and a soft, textured tunnel to intensify masturbation.

- **Cock ring** Worn at the base of the penis, these rings are designed to stiffen the erection and delay climax. Some have ears or studs on the upper side designed to stimulate the clitoris.
- **Cock and ball or Blakoe ring** Similar to a cock ring, this encircles the base of the penis and scrotum and is worn to give a sensation of tightness. Some have a strap that crosses the prostate and perineum (which might be ridged or studded) and is connected to a butt plug for maximum pleasure.
- **Sleeves** are designed to fit around the penis and can be covered in ridges, studs or bobbles for extra stimulation during penetration. Some come with a built-in ball ring.

Toy hints and tips

- You can learn more about your partner's masturbation technique by watching them use their toys.
- Some people like to have the tip of a toy inserted into the anus or vagina during oral play, or use one to stimulate the clitoris, testicles or prostate while having sex facing away from and astride their partner.
- Either put a fresh condom on your vibrator every time you use it or wash and dry it well after use before storing.
- ! Some people don't like sex toys. Never try to persuade anyone to try one against their will.

KINKS AND FETISHES

The terms kinks and fetishes are often used interchangeably – and there is some cross over – but they're very different things. Kelsey Borresen at *HuffPost* put it best: 'All fetishes are kinks, but not all kinks are fetishes'.

A kink refers to something that's an alternative or unusual sexual interest, preference or fantasy, although as sex is talked about more, and as sex positivity grows, it's harder to draw a line between usual and unusual and the adventurous. Spanking, hair pulling, breath play or role play would generally be considered kinks.

Fetishes, on the other hand, refer to objects or acts that are intrinsically linked to, or fundamental to, a person's sexual gratification. So if spanking or hair pulling was absolutely essential for sexual satisfaction in every sexual experience for someone, it wouldn't be called a kink and would instead be called a fetish.

Fetishes are often focused on a part of the body or an object that isn't overtly sexual. Foot fetishes are often the most talked about but others include noses, ankles, tickling, gravel or being dressed as a plush toy.

SAFE SPACE

There's still a lot of negativity towards kink and fetish play – intended or inadvertent – and it can make us anxious about exploring our own. But in a safe space and with someone you trust, it can be a really rewarding experience.

Some kinks will be a complete turn-off for some people but there shouldn't be any shame or embarrassment attached to sharing them. As always, communication and trust are key – talk first and if all parties are curious about something, discuss ways that you might ease yourselves in to putting them into practice. If someone just isn't into it, respect that and find other ways to enjoy play.

Fetishes can be more tricky to negotiate in all kinds of relationships. If your partner doesn't share your fetish, it may be hard for them to accept that they won't ever be able to completely satisfy you. Likewise, it might be very difficult for you to risk sharing something so deeply personal.

The kink and fetish communities are often incredibly open, welcoming and supportive of their members so spend time researching or chatting with people who share your needs or desires.

OTHER IDEAS

- It might sound vanilla but **read kinky stories**. EL James's *Fifty Shades of Grey* brought kink into the mainstream but erotic literature is a huge genre and there's plenty to inspire and arouse.
- Ever fancied literally **ripping** the clothes off your partner? Keep some old clothes specially for the purpose.
- In sex play, **body painting** can be used like a mask to release inhibitions and set a mood. It can inspire sex play, or it can be enjoyed just for itself – beautifying the body of your partner is an absorbing act of attention.
- Not just a word for suspenders, stockings and cut-out panties, **'lingerie'** is now a catch-all term for any underwear worn for its sex appeal. Slip or strap into something spicy made from mesh or chainmail; leather, latex or lace to play in an all new way. Use costume to explore fantasies – if you're unsure where to start think 'masked ball' or Moulin Rouge.
- Use **edging** to tease and tantalize your partner.
- A **swing** adds its own rhythm and gives an incredible sensation of near weightlessness. Consider fixing one up in your bedroom. The most crucial point is that the fixings should easily take both your weights and the momentum you generate, so you'll need a strong beam or joist on which to fix it.
- Watch porn together for arousal prior to or during play – it can enhance the experience or find new ideas and techniques to try.

EDGE-PLAY AND THE DANGERS OF EXTREMES

Edge-play describes any type of play that is significantly more risky than others, and almost all of it comes under the BDSM umbrella. Edge players might be putting themselves at increased risk of physical or psychological harm, or both, (or even death) as they are pushing themselves to their limits, and beyond.

Edge-play tests the limits of what consent really means and is dependent on both consent to non-consent, and risk awareness. Edge players are aware of the myriad risks involved and consent to activity that may realize that risk.

Among the most common forms of physical edge-play are electrosex (involving electricity), breath play (asphyxiation) and extreme insertions. But edge-play also includes things that involve a nihilistic element such as knowingly or willingly exposing yourself to infection or disease through unprotected sex with multiple partners or exchanging blood through cutting and blood play.

Edge-play is the most extreme form of sex and requires so much experience and nuance that we refuse to advocate for it in this book. However, it's a useful way in to explaining just how important boundaries and safety are before we discuss BDSM as even what is perceived as less-extreme BDSM play can put you at risk of physical, emotional and psychological harm.

Most forms of play can be adapted so that they sit on a spectrum of relatively safe to extremely dangerous.

- Bondage can be relatively safe if you are using bondage tape for short periods of time but extremely dangerous if you are suspended in ropes for long periods.
- Dripping molten wax across the body can be relatively safe but could also result in burns serious enough to require medical attention, or even permanent blindness.
- 'Choking' can be relatively safe if a hand is lightly cupped around a throat but extremely dangerous if pressure is applied and the air supply is cut off.
- Group sex with strangers can be relatively safe if protection is used but could result in contracting life-threatening diseases if protection is not used.

! Before entering any kind of play that has a BDSM element, identify the risks, set your own boundaries and be very, very sure that your playmate will respect them. If you're playing solo, ensure that you can call for immediate medical assistance if required.

BDSM

BDSM was once perceived as anything that wasn't considered normative, and often heteronormative. But today, it's really an umbrella term for anything that subverts power dynamics in sex play. Many of us will be enjoying kinks and techniques that would once have been called BDSM that we wouldn't recognize as such now.

In simple terms, BDSM breaks down like this:

- BD: Bondage and Discipline
- DS: Dominance and Submission
- SM: Sadism and Masochism

BDSM encompasses an almost endless variety of play, fun and fetishes on wildly varying scales of kink and pain. The only constant in BDSM play is that it is only ever consensual – if it isn't consensual, it's abuse.

Discipline, Humiliation and Degradation in Sex

Some people enjoy kinks such as Discipline, Humiliation and Degradation in their sex play. If you wish to explore these ideas, do your research first and take plenty of time to assess whether it might be right for you. Degradation and Humiliation require even more trust than other versions of the sub/dom dynamic and can leave you completely vulnerable and at yet further risk of harm.

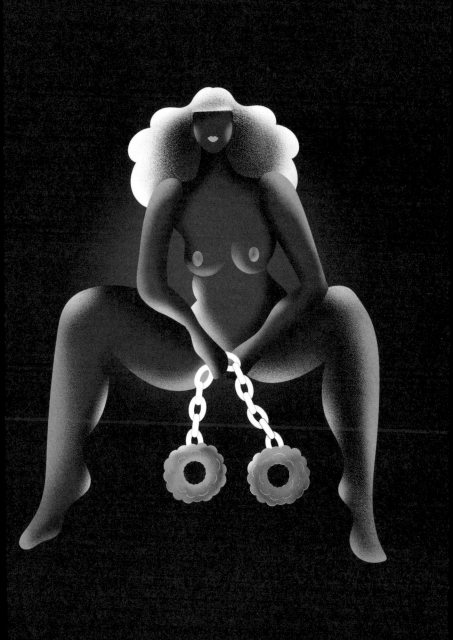

SUBMISSION AND DOMINANCE

Most people find something appealing in the idea of one partner being utterly at the mercy of the other. The submissive partner may be physically restrained in some way. The passive partner relinquishes responsibility, and is 'permitted' to enjoy what happens in a selfish way; the active partner takes full control, and this role too offers selfish pleasure, albeit of a different sort.

Fantasies of dominance and submission deny the mutual participation of the one-to-one adult sex act and, in making the two roles opposite and distinct, free the participants from the responsibilities of closeness. These fantasies may be acted out by couples who are shy of intimacy, and the release brought by acknowledging the different needs of each partner may paradoxically bring the couple closer together.

The thought of bondage, submission and dominance may seem weird – possibly even scary – to some, but for others it's merely a harmless and exciting way of exploring feelings they're denied in everyday life.

Playing a submissive (sub) or dominant (dom) role in sex can heighten your pleasure, allow you to turn fantasies into a reality and display traits that you can't otherwise exhibit. But introducing power dynamics into sex requires mutual respect, trust and clear boundaries.

What's in it for the dom? They get to do anything they like, and can have anything they like done to them. For the sub, it's a chance to relinquish responsibility for the sex act and explore aspects of sexuality that they might otherwise be too shy or embarrassed to try. It's also liberating in that it completely eliminates performance anxiety.

- If you're unsure of where to start, limit yourselves to 3 minutes of sub/dom play where the sub is the dom's sex doll.
- Or relinquish control of a remote-controlled vibrator to your partner.

NO PRESSURE

Communication is, as always, key. Make sure you're on the same page. If one of you is already into fetish play and your partner is unsure, it may help them to be reassured that you don't *need* it to be a part of sex but that you see it as an enhancement. Be prepared for them to refuse, and accept and respect that refusal.

Play by the rules

- Always discuss and plan in detail what you are going to do and how long it will last.
- Don't play when under the influence of drink or drugs.
- Never express or seek to arouse real anger and aggression.

BONDAGE

Bondage is a first step into the world of sub/dom play. If you're new to it, or not ready for ropes and chains, gently bind the wrists with stockings or scarves with arms extended above the head. Then experiment with the wrists bound behind your back. There are beginners' bondage kits available and many use bondage tape – a skin-friendly alternative to ropes and cords.

BEFORE YOU TIE UP YOUR PARTNER

! Never tie anyone up against their will.

! Being bound leaves people incredibly vulnerable – check in with them regularly to ensure they are emotionally and physically comfortable.

! Use safe ties. Don't do anything that will cut off air supply or circulation. Don't use slip knots, as they tighten when pulled. Always check that you can slip two fingers between your partner's skin and the rope – if you can't, the rope is too tight.

! Don't leave anyone alone once you have bound them up.

! Agree on a safe word before you start – don't use the word 'no' – and always end the game immediately if you hear it. Safety words don't suggest inherent danger; they're used to ensure participants can relax safe in the knowledge that they can stop at any time without their words being misconstrued. Similarly, always agree on boundaries and be confident in setting rules such as no anal, no spanking.

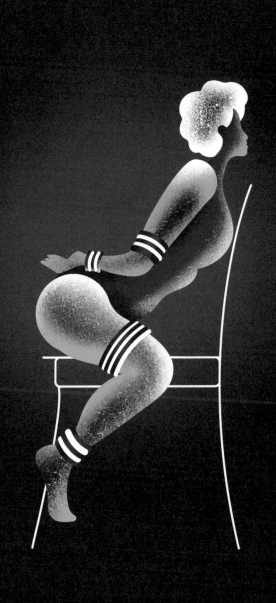

How to Tie

- **Chair tie**. Sit your partner on a chair, their bum as close to the edge of the seat as possible with legs apart. Tie their left ankle to the left chair leg, then repeat for the right leg. Take their hands behind their backs and tie the wrists together, then tie their wrists to the back of the chair. Or, have them straddle the chair backwards, bum facing out, arms bound to the backrest, ankles tied to the chair legs.
- **Hog tie**. Best for submissive partners with upper body and spinal flexibility. Lay them face down, legs apart. Raise their ankles until they're above the buttocks and tie the ankles together. Bring their wrists together and down towards the buttocks and tie the wrists together. Then tie the bound ankles to the bound wrists.
- **Frog tie**. Best for partners with flexible hips and legs. Lie them on their back with legs apart, knees bent. Tie around their left thigh, then their left calf and then tie the left thigh to the left calf. Repeat for the right leg.

PLEASURE AND PAIN

Pleasure and pain frequently overlap as both stimulate the amygdala – a part of the brain associated with reward.

IMPACT PLAY

Smacking, slapping, flogging and whipping are all forms of impact play. Impact play is incredibly arousing and can enhance the intensity of orgasm.

- Slap the buttocks with short, hard slaps with a hand or paddle. Pause between slaps until your partner feels a tingle or burn and slowly increase the intensity and frequency.
- Slap breasts and chests with short, sharp crosswise slaps that graze the nipple.
- Flick the clitoris or nipples with one or two fingers with short, sharp flicks. This is enjoyable in itself but can also prepare you for the sensation of flogging and whipping.
- Flogging is more suitable for beginners than whipping. A flog has multiple fronds and, if used correctly, is often less painful. Choose a soft flog with no studs or knotted ends. Avoid sensitive areas such as the shoulders, breasts, lower legs and genitals – start with the back or buttocks and make very precise and gentle strokes. Pause for 3–7 seconds between strokes. Avoid the ends of the flog wrapping around more sensitive areas – if you're flogging the upper back, ensure the ends aren't going to strike the rib cage. Only once you've perfected the art of using the flog, and your partner consents, should you move on to other areas of the body.

There needn't be an overt sub/dom or sado masochistic element to play that involves pleasure and pain – it can be just as exciting as part of adventurous, neutral play.

TEMPERATURE PLAY

A sensual play that involves stimulation with extremes of temperature. Some like it hot, some like it cold, some like switching between the two.

Cold

- Hold an ice cube in your mouth before nipple play or oral sex. You can brush your partner's skin with your cold lips and tongue, or gently push the ice cube against it. Lay the ice cube on their pubic bone or chest and allow it to melt and run across their body.
- Fill a condom with water and freeze it. Once frozen, it can be used as a wand or dildo.
- ❗ Always run ice cubes or wands briefly under cold water so that it doesn't stick to or burn the skin.

Hot

- Drip and drizzle molten candle wax across each other's bodies. Some candles melt into massage oils while others harden on the skin – for some people, having the wax peeled off is all part of the pleasure.

- Start slow and focus on the back, down the arms and across the buttocks or thighs. A slow, steady drip can build anticipation quickly, or a short, sharp drizzle can deliver a burst of pleasure.
- Use a 'body safe' candle and always avoid the eyes, genitals and open wounds. Drip and drizzle the wax slowly and from a height to avoid burns – we recommend a distance of 15 inches. If you use a massage candle, be aware that the natural oils will break down condoms so wash hands and bodies thoroughly before handling them.

BREATH PLAY

Breath play (or asphyxiation) involves restricting a body's air supply in order to heighten arousal. Some people love the light-headedness that comes with asphyxiation, and the rush of blood that comes as the choke is released. But breath play is inherently dangerous (and frequently fatal) and is a no-go area for us.

SAFETY

There is a clear line between unwanted pain and pleasurable pain and exploring rough or dominant play is not a licence for cruelty. If you're playing sub/dom roles, the dom is responsible for ensuring that the sub is safe, comfortable and experiencing pleasure at all times. If there is no pleasure and only pain, stop immediately.

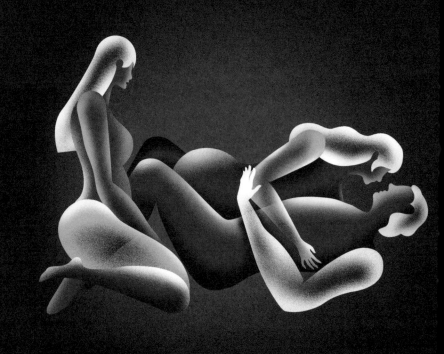

GROUP SEX

Group play or group sex is a common fantasy but is practised less frequently than others. That's partly because group sex is an age-old taboo that until relatively recently, wasn't talked about outside of shamey documentaries; partly because group sex can be a difficult subject to raise with a partner – particularly in committed relationships; and partly because it can expose you to a host of dangers and risks.

There are many reasons group play appeals to people. First up is the obvious – in a group, you're increasing your opportunities for arousal and stimulation by sheer numbers. There are more mouths and more hands on you, more orifices to explore and more to see, smell, taste and hear. For others, they find themselves more able to be truly sexually free. Some people find that being in a committed relationship, or playing with just one partner, can limit what they're able to explore. Anonymity, or an element of emotional detachment, removes those limitations and they feel less self-conscious about fulfilling their own needs and desires.

WATCHING

Group sex doesn't necessarily mean you need to engage in play with anyone, or anyone other than your partner. It can be an opportunity to reveal your inner-exhibitionist, or simply enjoy the experience of being the watcher. Being a witness to intimate, real-world sex can be a powerfully moving and erotic experience that bears no comparison to watching porn or professional acts in a sex club.

- If you've decided to invite someone or someones to join you for the first time, at least one of you is bound to feel awkward – particularly if it's everyone's first group experience.
- If you've decided to have group sex because you've watched porn, read our page on porn first because real-life group sex is often a totally different experience to what you see on screen (as is true of almost all play!). There's going to be more awkward manoeuvring into new positions and more of the potentially embarrassing bits. Communicate. And laugh.
- Threesomes can be trickier to negotiate for beginners or new groups as it's easy to create a third wheel. Make sure no one is left out of the fun.

EVENTS, CLUBS AND PARTIES

There is an increasing number of regular events and nights that cater to everyone, and ones that place participants' safety above all else. Do your research and check the event rules – the best events will clearly advertise them and be wary of any that don't.

Often, people find that attending an event is the most simple route to exploring group sex. It can be embarrassing, difficult and risky to invite a mutual friend or acquaintance to play, and if you're unsure what the effect on a relationship might be, going to a night where you're guaranteed anonymity, and don't have to play with anyone else, eases those worries.

GROUPS AND RELATIONSHIPS

Once upon a time, 'swinging' was called 'wife swapping'
– a deeply problematic and toxic term. We've all come
a long way since then and 'swinging' is now something
that couples of any gender participate in, and everyone
involved is an equal.

Some couples introduce group play into their relationships to
add spice, and experience pleasures and kinks that they may
not otherwise be able to share or act out on one another.

If you're in a relationship, group sex can enhance your
attraction to and appreciation of your partner, and your
mutual pleasure. As always, talk to your partner first. Consider
what you're each looking for, what you hope to gain, what you
might like to try. Exploring possible scenarios together can
build anticipation well in advance.

Group play requires mutual respect and trust, and both
partners to be able to agree to physical and emotional
boundaries ahead of time. In committed relationships, it's
common to set boundaries on 'intimacy' such as no kissing,
no cuddling, no breaking away from the group to find
somewhere private.

! It's not for everyone and is rarely a positive solution
  in relationships where there is jealousy, betrayal,
  unhappiness or dissatisfaction.

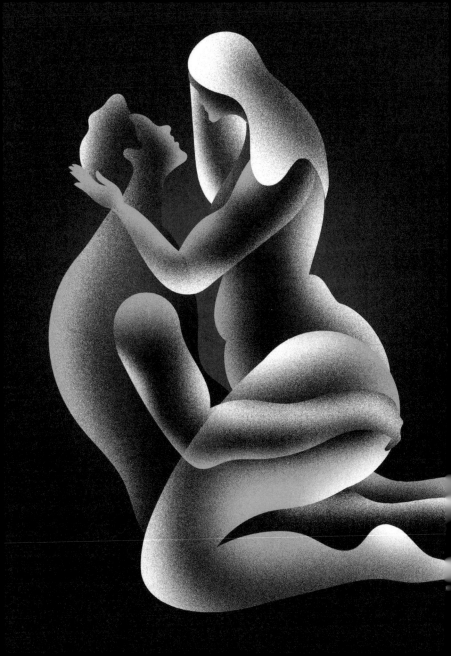